Spirituality, Healing and Medicine

of related interest

Music Therapy Research and Practice in Medicine
From Out of the Silence
David Aldridge
ISBN 1 85302 296 9

Music Therapy in Palliative Care
New Voices
Edited by David Aldridge
ISBN 1 85302 739 1

Suicide
The Tragedy of Hopelessness
David Aldridge
ISBN 1 85302 444 9

Spirituality and Ageing
Edited by Albert Jewell
ISBN 1 85302 631 X

Spirituality in Mental Health Care
John Swinton
ISBN 1 85302 804 5

Spiritual Dimensions of Pastoral Care
Practical Theology in a Multidisciplinary Context
Edited by David Willows and John Swinton
ISBN 1 85302 892 4

Spirituality, Healing and Medicine

Return to the Silence

David Aldridge

Jessica Kingsley Publishers
London and Philadelphia

The right of David Aldridge to be identified as author of this work has been asserted by him in accordance with the Copyright, Designs and Patents Act 1988.

First published in the United Kingdom in 2000 by
Jessica Kingsley Publishers Ltd
116 Pentonville Road
London N1 9JB, England
and
325 Chestnut Street,
Philadelphia, PA19106, USA

www.jkp.com

Library of Congress Cataloging in Publication Data
Aldridge, David
    Spirituality, healing and medicine : return to silence / David Aldridge
        p. cm
    Includes bibliographical references and index.
    ISBN 1 85302 554 2 (alk. paper)
    1. Spiritual healing. 2. Medicine-- Religious aspects. 1. Title.
BL65.M4.A53 2000
615.8'52--dc21   99-087312

British Library Cataloguing in Publication Data
A CIP catalogue record for this book is available from the British Library

ISBN 1 85302 554 2 pb

Printed and Bound in Great Britain by
Athenaeum Press, Gateshead, Tyne and Wear

Contents

List of Figures and Tables

Figures

Tables

This book is dedicated to Irina Tweedie (1907–1999)

Acknowledgements

I would like to thank Gudrun for the necessary patience required for living with an author.

Vibeke Steffen made an important contribution in bringing her knowledge of medical anthropology, her understanding of working with alcoholics and her encouragement to make a start on the text.

Through the years, kind comments of support from Dan Benor, Daniel Wirth, Kim Jobst, Harris Dienstfrey and Larry Dossey have reminded me that there are others out there pursuing the same elusive knowledge.

Lutz Neugebauer and Susan Weber kept asking when the book would be finished so they could read it and this has kept me dedicated to my readership of at least two.

Finally, I would like to thank my mother who lends her only copy of a former book of mine, now out of print, to friends in her church. Hopefully, this one too will find a suitable purpose.

Comment

I have used as little capitalization of god, divine and church as possible. No offence is meant by this. It is simply to avoid the appearance of a Victorian religious tract. Where a particular Church or a belief in God is referred to, then I use capitals. The use of he and she is applied randomly throughout for the gender of patients, healers or doctors, unless necessary to the context.

1

Healing narratives in the context of a performed life

Our spirit is the real part of us, our body its garment. A man would not find peace at the tailor's because his coat comes from there: neither can the spirit obtain true happiness from the earth just because his body belongs to earth. (Inayat Khan 1979)

The very fact of our existence is a prayer and compelling – 'I am, therefore I pray – sum ergo oro.' It is a quality of the Divine basis of existence while acknowledging our temporal material existence. (Frithjof Schuon 1989)

The natural science base of modern medicine, which in turn influences the way in which modern medicine is delivered, often ignores the spiritual factors associated with health. Health invariably becomes defined in anatomical or physiological, psychological or social terms. Rarely do we find diagnoses which include the relationship between the patient and their God. The descriptions we invoke have implications for the treatment strategies we suggest, the way in which we understand how people can be encouraged to become healthy and the policies that we implement to maintain that state which we call 'health'. Patience, grace, prayer, meditation, hope, forgiveness and fellowship are as important in many of our health initiatives as medication, hospitalization, or surgery. The spiritual elements of experience help us to rise above the matters at hand such that in the face of suffering we can find purpose, meaning and hope. It is in the understanding of suffering, the universality of suffering and the need for deliverance from it that varying traditions of medicine and religion meet.

Important changes have been taking place in both the church and within medicine. Issues relating to health and well-being have been raised that question the fundamental practices of these institutions. Principally these issues are about the definition of health and who is to be involved in healing. These issues are not new and are raised at times of transformation when the old order, whether it be in church or medicine, is being challenged. To make a challenge is both to claim and to accuse. It can also mean to invite or summon, to call into question, to make demands on, and is a call to engage in some sort of activity. This is what I am trying to do in this book: to challenge the reader to engage in talking about spirituality. I am aware that the word challenge is also related to the Latin *caluminia*, the word we know as calumny, which is to make a false claim. Indeed, as soon as we talk about being spiritual, particularly in terms of healing, then we are prey to hubris and the possibility of making claims for something that we perhaps do not possess. Indeed, the claim of being able to heal by lay practitioners is certain to inflame those practitioners licensed by the state. But our expectations of modern medicine can also lead us to overreach ourselves. We promise to deliver a technology which frees us from disease, yet we know that those claims are partial. Chronic diseases are still a challenge. Mental health problems are recalcitrant.

What is important to make clear from the very beginning is that I am not proposing spiritual healing as an alternative to modern health-care delivery. Modern medicine and its complementary forms are the basis of health-care delivery in the Western industrialized nations (Aldridge 1990b). What I am arguing for is that within this pluralistic system of health-care delivery we accept that some patients and practitioners will want to express their understandings of health, illness, recovery and treatment in terms which are spiritual, as well as physical, psychological and social. Further, some patients and practitioners will want to participate in forms of healing that include spiritual considerations within a pluralistic context of modern health-care delivery.

There is a growing demand by health-care consumers for involvement in health-care issues and for initiatives promoting a healthy lifestyle. Within the church too there are demands by the laity to be actively involved in the life of the church and for lay ministries to be recognized. Communities are eager to make decisions about matters which affect their daily lives and are no longer willing to abdicate the sole process of decision making to licensed and expert professionals who may be far removed from them in terms of educational background, social class and experience. This does not mean that there is a revolt against expert health advice from health professionals or the clergy. What is proposed is that these experts become facilitators and informed advisers within a system of health-care deliverers, providers and consumers. What we appear to be seeing is that in wealthy industrialized nations, where basic health-care needs are satisfied, health appears as a commodity linked not to the survival needs of fresh water and drainage but to existential needs. This is not to say that health-care needs are not threatened by the pollution of those basic services, but the problem is one of glut rather than poverty.

George

The case of my friend George, who had leukaemia, pulls together many of the paths I will explore in this book. His parish priest asked me to visit him in hospital (Aldridge 1987c). We discussed hypnosis, at his initiation, as a means of pain management and for strengthening his resolve. I gave him a pre-recorded meditation tape to prepare him for the sound of my voice and as a precursor to any therapeutic interventions. Ironically, under the pressure of need, he used it within the first few days to gain rest and sleep within the context of a busy hospital ward and between varying medical procedures (his bone marrow was removed, treated and replaced). From this basis, we developed a set of visualizations that encouraged him to experience the flow of healing within him and methods which he could use in facing his various difficulties and challenges (the struggle to carry on after the exhaustion of hospital treatment, to survive the various rounds of hospital visits, tests and overcome the worry of daily living). These interventions were psychological and social. At the same time the specialist dealing with cancers of the blood was making interventions, filtering and transplanting blood cells, which were biomedical. His priest prayed for him and counselled him. His wife encouraged him to keep up his fighting spirit for her sake and for his two sons.

What we did, priest, psychologist, patient, spouse and physician, was to co-operate in our approaches. We were trying, in the light of the failing medical interventions, to develop an ecology of treatment at various levels, physical, psychological, social and spiritual, which would meet the needs of George and his family. The cancer specialist responsible for the medical treatment knew that George needed something more than he could give, even though he was working to the limit of his technical abilities. What the oncologist knew was that, although technology was failing us, hope was an important factor for George. As a clinician he knew that although his scientific and technological resources were exhausted, there were other healing resources within the community. This was *diagnosis* in the broadest sense of the term, knowledge based not solely upon physiology but upon the deep needs of the patient and his family. Neither knowledge excluded the other; both were reconciled in who George was, in his personal need. From this basis, a *prognosis* could be made. George would die. But 'How would he die?' was the question we all were asking.

At the same time there were regular sessions of prayer, the laying on of hands and a celebration of the Christian eucharist at George's home. Family and friends from near and far were invited to visit. Some wanted to 'lay on hands' and pray directly for George, even though they, like George and his family, had not experienced such healing practice before. The symbolic act of 'reaching out' was important for their understanding. In this sense healing is a sacrament, an outer sign of something that is hidden. The reaching out of a friend, for George, was the reaching out of God to heal; to heal, not necessarily to cure. This is the significance of the sacrament of the laying on of hands as a sacred reality (Csordas 1983) and not to be equated as some writers do with the therapeutic touch of the doctor as a secular reality.

George was dying and, as he said, literally living on the blood of others. For him, this sacrifice of blood from human donors and the celebration of the blood and body of Christ with bread and wine took on a powerful spiritual meaning. His friends too were affected by the resonance of an ancient sacrament within the setting of a modern medical intervention. Medicine was enlivened by a symbolic understanding. From the technological act of transfusion there was a transformation of understanding that blood literally was given for him that he may have life. This is both the literal and the metaphoric together and is a powerful expression of unified meaning. I shall return to this argument of the literal and metaphoric later in discussing the concept of 'energy' in healing. It is also the instrumental reason for spiritual understandings, not an evidential display of healing; instrumental in that, through this act of donorship, another awareness was promoted. All involved were challenged to understand the meaning of sacrament in a real way.

Death as an outcome of living

Eventually George died at home in the arms of his wife with his children beside him. Our treatment failed yet we, psychologist, priest and physician, believed he was healed. In terms of health outcomes we had failed. Yet the manner in which he had died and the ramifications for those with whom the process of dying had taken place could be considered as a positive resolution. George had suffered, and suffered terribly. We had all taken part in trying to relieve that suffering, with success and failure. However, in that suffering and its palliation George found peace and reconciliation. Friends, family and physician found comfort and meaning within the context of dying that extended the best of our human capabilities.

When we talk of contexts for healing we all too often concentrate on patients in terms of a narrow range of healing outcome narratives. Yet we have to see the ramifications for those who survive and the way in which treatment or success take their toll on the practitioners involved. While the physician must endeavour to maintain life, in the context of those others who are involved in patient care and the patient himself, then death must not necessarily be seen as a negative outcome. I am not arguing here for euthanasia, rather in the long-term interests of my medical colleagues. Part of the contract of accepting life, which we make at conception, is that this corporeal existence will come to an end. Both life and death are part of the same contract. While we strive to bring lives to their fullness and maintain lives to their intended span, if we see death always as a negative outcome then we burden ourselves with an unnecessary suffering. Part of this expectation stems from a modern scientific perspective that, in its triumphalist technology, expects to conquer nature. It is this very displacement from an ecological understanding, accepting both birth and death in the longer cycle of life, that is causing further suffering.

Health as narrative performance: A developing theme

This book is the third of three related titles, the first of which is about music therapy in the practice of medicine (Aldridge 1996). The first book proposes an alternative metaphor for understanding human beings. Rather than seeing ourselves as mechanical beings, constructed like machines and obeying strict causal laws, it is argued that we are in a continual state of improvisation, like music. We are beings with identities continually in performance; symphonic beings rather than mechanical objects. There is an aesthetic that governs our lives. It is an attempt to explain how music therapy can bring about change within the individual, unifying both mind and body. While we often use the injunction 'I think, therefore I am', the argument may be better expressed as 'I perform, therefore I am'. In this sense health too is a performed activity; a performance that takes place with others and, while dependent upon the body, incorporates mind and spirit. It is this very incarnation of the psychic, cultural and spiritual that is the crux of the following arguments. Rather than deny the body, as some religious movements do, or reify the body alone, as scientific medicine often does, I shall be arguing here in Chapter 4 that the body is the place of a performed praxis aesthetic of health care embodying that which we call spiritual.

In some ways it appears that the Church has retained the soul and medicine the body. What is needed is a reunification of both, where soul and body are seen as interpretations of the same phenomena.

The principal argument from the first book is that our lives are dynamic and performed in defining contexts that lend them meaning. The context of life in the cell will be the organ, the context for the organ will be the body, that of the body will be the 'environment'. This environment may indeed be the physical environment; it will also be a social environment, a broader ecological environment of nature but also an environment of ideas. It is this ecology of ideas that is profoundly important for being human and reflects human consciousness. We are influenced by the landscape of consciousness in which we have our being. However, I am not arguing for idealism but a transformation of consciousness, which will demand a compassionate acceptance of the material world as it relates to an understanding of the spiritual.

In the second book, concerning suicide (Aldridge 1998), the tragedy of hopelessness that we face as an existential landscape in our modern industrial communities is discussed. Where the first book was concerned with a performed identity, this second book is concerned with how those performed lives gain their

TN14411

meaning in interaction and the interpretation of events. In this sense, identity is performed in various social arenas with a variety of purposive actors that lend meaning to what is performed. Culture is an ecological activity binding the meanings of individuals in relationships together, what Gregory Bateson (1972) refers to as an 'ecology of mind' (discussed in the next chapter). What we do as individuals is understood in the setting of our social activities and those settings are informed by the individuals that comprise them (Browner 1998). Here too, the body and the presentation of symptoms are seen as an important non-verbal communication that has meaning within specific personal relationships which are located themselves within a social context. Symptoms are interpreted within relationships.

While non-verbal communication features in both books, a central plank of the argument in the book about suicide is the importance of the story the patient and his or her family relate about the problems they face; not simply the story itself, but the way the story is told. A patient's narrative about his illness does not point out the meaning directly, it demonstrates meaning by recreating pattern in metaphorical shape or form in the telling that is interpreted within relationship. Symptoms here are a symbolic communication as they are told and confessed. Symptoms are signs that have to be both observed and interpreted in their performance. Stories give a sense of pattern, a way of speaking, perceiving and existing, whereas concepts tend to nominalize. Our task is not to impose a meaning on the story but to allow its meaning to become manifest in relationship with the teller. Narratives are constructed and interpreted. They lend meaning to what happens in daily life. We all have our biographies. What happens to our bodies is related to our identities as persons. These narratives are not simply personal constructions but negotiated in the contexts of our intimate relation-ships. These understandings are also constructed within a cultural context that lends legitimacy to those narratives. Thus meanings are nested within a hierarchy of contexts. The same process applies to the history of our bodies, to the biography of our selves, to the narratives used by healers, or to the tales told by the elders of a tribe.

What I try to do in both books is to show that meanings are linked to actions, and those actions have consequences that are performed. What our patients think about the causes of their illnesses will influence what they do in terms of treatment, which in turn will influence what they do in the future. As practitioners, we lend meaning to the events that are related to us by our patients, weaving them into the fabric of our treatment strategies. For suicidal patients, if those causes and consequences are at odds with what the practitioner finds acceptable, then there is the potential for escalating distress. I argue that we must learn to understand each other's language for expressing and resolving distress, and act consequently. That this language may be non-verbal and predicated upon bodily expression returns me once more to a praxis aesthetic. It is the hanged body, the poisoned corpse, the mutilated torso, with which we are presented as a representation of psychic distress where human spirit has failed to maintain life to its expected fullness. Suffering is embodied as pain. While we may temporarily relieve pain with analgesics, our task is also to understand and thereby relieve suffering. In this way the ecology of ideas, that some call knowledge, is explicated within the body as a correspondence between mental representations and the material world.

This third book is a synthesis. It is an existential account of what it is to perform health, how that performed health is dependent upon a variety of negotiated meanings and how those meanings are transcended. As human beings we continue to develop. Body and self are narrative constructions, stories that are related to intimates at chosen moments. These meanings are concerned with body, mind and spirit. My intention is to set about the task of reviving a set of meanings given to the understanding of human behaviour that is termed spiritual. What I would like to establish is that it is legitimate to talk about spirituality in a culture of health-care delivery. To achieve this I shall collate documentary material from varying disciplines. In talking about suicide, an ecological approach was adopted to understand how human beings perform their lives together in meaningful contexts of significant others that are nested within broader social contexts. This book too extends that ecological understanding and will argue for a return to a sacred understanding of human beings and nature. In these instances, 'God', 'the divine', 'the cosmos' or 'nature' may be the name given to a meaningful immanent context in which life is performed.

Spiritual meanings are linked to actions, and those actions have consequences that are performed as prayer, meditation, worship and healing. What patients think about the causes of their illnesses influences what they do in terms of health-care treatment and to whom they turn for the resolution of distress. For some people, rather than consider illness alone, they relate their personal identities to being healthy, one factor of which is spirituality. The maintenance and promotion of health, or becoming healthy, is an activity. As such it will be expressed bodily, a praxis aesthetic. Thus we would expect to see people not only having sets of beliefs about health but also actions related to those beliefs. Some of these may be dietary, some involve exercise and some prayer or meditation. In more formal terms they may wish to engage in spiritual healing and contact a spiritual healer among the health-care practitioners whom they consult. Indeed, some medical practitioners refer patients to spiritual healers.

There is no intent in this book to develop a strong argument for the practice of spiritual healing, although I shall use some of the relevant literature. Nor will there be any attempt to put forward a detailed and comprehensive argument for each and every direction in spiritual healing. Such an endeavour has been better accomplished by specialist authors (Benor 1990; Benor 1991; Benor 1992;

Dossey 1993; Wirth 1995; Wirth *et al.* 1993; Wirth *et al.* 1996a; Wirth and Cram 1997; Wirth, Richardson and Eidelman 1996b). The approach here will be to take examples from pertinent areas of research where spirituality is mentioned. From talking with a variety of health-care practitioners, their requirement is for examples of what spirituality in health care is so that they can grasp what is being proposed. Each of the following chapters will take a particular theme and expand upon it as it relates to health care based on the diversity of available literature.

In addition, as the languages used to describe spiritual healing are so varied, it is necessary to offer bridges between various understandings. Talking about spiritual healing and active considerations of spirituality can enter even the most traditional medical forum (Aldridge 1991a, 1991c; Carey 1997), but the language must be chosen carefully. While modern scientific medicine may be gradually opening to such ideas, the church may be sometimes closed to such understanding. Larry Dossey, for example, has been influential as a medical practitioner for promoting the value of prayer, yet he has been criticized by churchgoers for his support of psi phenomena. Similarly, a Christian bishop in an English cathedral at a celebration of healing ministries criticized any members of the congregation who showed interest in traditional Chinese medicine as it imported an 'Eastern spirituality'. Not only did this alienate people who had come from far and wide, in the spirit of hope, to hear of reconciliation within a healing movement, but it also expressed a narrow chauvinism of Western thought that exiled more than it included. Presumably Bethlehem and the Galilean hinterland are a part of the English home counties.

Raising consciousness, realizing truth

By spirituality I am talking about the refining of human consciousness in reaching the truth. While many practitioners accept the use of subconscious causes, physiological demands and biological drives as lower levels of consciousness, it is difficult to bring into a scientific discussion that there are varying levels of consciousness which human beings can achieve and some of these are higher, or at least more subtle, than those that we currently have. I shall not be denying bodily awareness, simply reinstating such awareness within defining contexts of consciousness. This is surely the basis of perception, which I refer to as systemic ecology. These contexts of consciousness are nested one within another, but the influence is not simply that of higher orders determining lower orders but also that lower processes will constrain higher processes. Thus bodily techniques of breathing can influence consciousness, as we see in meditation. Similarly, ideas about the meaning of life and the purpose of living can also have significant effects upon physiological parameters, as we see in chronic heart disease.

Definitions of spirituality, as they occur in the literature, will be made later in Chapter 2. For those readers who would remind me that we have science as the basis of truth claims, the argument here, as in the previous two books, is that art and theology are also purveyors of truths within our civilized cultures and have contributions to make to the healing debate. That science alone, as realized in technology, is used as the overriding argument for understanding modern living, is for some the cause of modern problems. Technology divorced from ethics leads to an unbalanced ecology. The inclusion of various discourses other than science is not an argument against science, rather that science be placed within a cultural domain alongside other truth claims.

What we have to ask, as health-care practitioners is whether the inclusion of spirituality brings advantages to understanding the people who come to us in distress. As soon as we talk about life being something to cherish and preserve, that compassion for others plays an important role in the way in which we choose to live with each other, that service to our communities is a vital activity for maintaining well-being, that hope is an important factor in recovery, then we have the basis for an argument that is spiritual as well as scientific. Essentially I am arguing for a plurality of understanding in terms of sickness and healing. How do we make meaningful connections that form the narratives we make as patients and practitioners and how do those narratives inform each other? While we may have expert technologies of healing, we cannot divorce those technologies from the ethics of health-care delivery.

Understanding each other

Our stories are our identities. How we relate them to each other constructively, so that we mutually understand each other, is the basis of communication. What we do, or persuade others to do, as a consequence of those communicated stories is an exercise of power. While we may have sophisticated instruments of communication for transferring data as information, the digital technologies of cellular telephone networks and the 'web', how we understand the meanings of others cannot be so easily achieved. Delivering data is no problem; understanding each other demands another level of involvement that is simply not technical.

We shall also see, in Chapter 4, that people are focusing on achieving health, rather than on becoming ill. Thus we enter a domain that is not practitioner bound. Consumers are making specific and informed demands of the expert practitioner and of the market that supplies health care. Of these health-care activities, an orientation to the future, that links with the past and is achieved in the present, will be based not only on understandings but practices related to those understandings. If hope is an understanding of the future realized now, in the present, then we have a practical understanding of a spiritual activity. Hope is a common term in our culture that appears to be acceptable to scientists, priests and laity. Hope, while based on belief, becomes manifest in action. What we do is as important as what we think and understand. Both are related. As I discussed in the second of these three related books, suicide is the tragedy of hopelessness. Promoting hope will be a significant endeavour in living fully and expressed in what we do.

There are different methods to approach truth. If we accept that in a modern vibrant culture there is a pluralism of truth claims, then a major task will be for us to reconcile what may appear to be disparate ideas. The argument here is not for some kind of homogeneity of thought but for an acceptance of the tension between ideas as a creative arena that pushes us beyond what we know. Thomas Merton (1966) writes in his journal for 28 April 1957:

> If I can unite in myself, in my own spiritual life, the thought of the East and West of the Greek and Latin fathers, I will create in myself a reunion of the divided Church and from that unity in myself can come the exterior and visible unity of the Church. For if we want to bring together East and West we cannot do it by imposing one upon the other. We must contain both within ourselves and transcend both. (Merton 1966, p.87)

My hope is that within this book we can go some way to uniting the 'East' and 'West' of thinking in spirituality and science such that there is a reunion of thought about healing and the possibility of transcendence. This perhaps is the basis of healing and the core of hope. As Merton suggests, one cannot be imposed upon the other; it is the containment within ourselves that brings the change. That is why I am at pains to remind the reader that this is not an evangelical tract for spiritual healing, simply an argument for diversity in the culture of health care that includes the spiritual. In the same vein, I am not arguing against modern health-care delivery or scientific methods, but for the development of an applied knowledge that relieves suffering and promotes tolerance.

Knowledge gained

At the heart of our understanding of the world is knowledge. If there are various ways to the truth, then there are varying ways to achieve knowledge. What we know influences what we do. What we do influences the way in which knowledge is acquired. While modern medical science is predicated upon empiricism and knowledge through the senses, there is another source of knowledge through contemplation and meditation. The plea of this book is that both reason and intuition be considered. In a world where often loud aggressive activity appears to be the most convincing evidence of personal surety, then the knowledge that comes from out of the silence may appear to have little influence. But it is to this knowledge that we may have to return; it is from here that the soul cries out to us in its suffering. If gnosis is the source of knowing, then for the future of our health-care endeavours we may have to broaden the sources of knowledge to include both the scientific and the spiritual in a reconciliation that is complementary. From such a reconciled basis of knowledge, we can enrich both *diagnosis* and *prognosis*.

Perhaps an example from clinical practice will illustrate what the inclusion of spirituality may bring for the benefit of the patient.

Eva

A woman came to see me in distress. She was referred by her general practitioner who was concerned for her mental state. Her husband had recently died. She had become suicidal and my task at that time was to research into suicidal behaviour. As she talked about what had happened over the previous year, it became increasingly clear that the woman had faced a series of tragedies in her life leaving her increasingly alone and distressed. However, both in the way that she talked about her problems concerning those varying life events and in the symptoms she presented, there seemed to be no obvious elements of mental illness. Nor did my psychiatrist colleague find any such signs. On asking Eva about what the central problem was, she said it was that she had lost her relationship with her God. Her husband was dead, her family estranged, her body was failing her and she saw no reason to live. These were all signs for her that God had abandoned her.

This presented me with a dilemma because instead of the conversation staying within a predictable framework of life events and symptoms, or even florid descriptions of a supernatural world, the woman sitting before me was giving a clear account of an existential world that had lost its meaning. Her purpose for living had gone: not solely in the loss of her husband, which had been a massive blow in itself, but in the sequelae of that loss. The question remained about how to approach this problem. Surely she needed a priest, not a research psychologist? Here lay the crux of the dilemma. Whenever she had talked about the nature of her problem as the loss of her relationship with God, that living made no sense to her, she was either passed on as mentally unstable by her general practitioner, who like me felt unable to locate her problem within his own sphere of competence, or misunderstood by the priest who prescribed prayer. Either she was stigmatized, in her eyes, by her doctor, or she was asked to do something impossible, to pray, by the priest.

In a previous book (Aldridge 1998) I have described this escalation of distress and how it may be compounded by the cycle of attempted resolutions, in this case referral or prayer. Referral to a psychologist and psychiatric services was seen by her as an act of rejection and humiliation. In her own eyes she was not crazy but suffering. Her priest offered a solution that was as untenable as being labelled mentally ill. He asked her to pray to a God in whom she no longer believed, in a church where she no longer felt at home, and before a symbol of the crucifixion that both reflected and exacerbated her suffering. Fortunately I had trained with a colleague who had left the priesthood in a crisis of faith and became a social worker. He offered to talk with her and, despite another referral, she eventually found a partner with whom she could begin to make sense of her existence in spiritual terms, but without the confines of a religious context.

We see here how distress can be manifested in a way that finds no immediate resolution within the framework of health-care delivery. The woman was using a language about a spiritual need for which those of us in the various helping agencies had no vocabulary other than that of a potential pathology. Yet this language is perfectly legitimate within a broader cultural context. In terms of her distress, where was she to find healing? Both bastions of culture, medicine and the church, were failing her in that we were deaf to the language in which she was expressing her dilemma. This book is about how that language can be revived, how legitimacy can be restored to the notion of spirituality within our health-care endeavours.

While conventional religions are intended as vehicles for the teaching and expression of spirituality, this book will also attempt to understand spirituality as understandings that may not always be located in religious contexts. Eva was undergoing a crisis of faith, albeit presented in somatic and psychological symptoms to her general practitioner. No amount of medication was going to resolve this crisis. But a counsellor who understood the crisis of faith and the dark night of the soul could offer her a way to find resolution. Practitioners and researchers are not being asked to abandon the language of natural science, but simply to accept that within our varying cultures there are complementary vocabularies and repertoires of healing which have their own validity and with which those people who come to us as sufferers narrate the performance of their own lives. To deny the validity of their language of expression as it is performed in the dramaturgy of their lives is to deny legitimacy to the identity of the sufferer, which contributes further to the suffering (Aldridge 1998).

Narrative regained

We will see in Chapter 4 that health is a praxis aesthetic, the performed body located in social relationship belonging to a culture of shared understandings. Spirituality is seen as a change in consciousness brought about by ritual. Religion is the social context that offers forms of understanding and practice that are made specific by culture. Spirituality brings about changes in consciousness that are transcendental and achieved through a higher power or connection with a greater unity. Such changes of consciousness, embedded in the social and embodied in the individual, bring about changes in health. The social is incorporated literally 'in the body' and that incorporation is transcended through changes in consciousness, which become themselves incarnate. Through the body we have articulations of distress and health. While health may be concerned with the relief of distress and can also be performed for its own sake, sickness is a separate phenomenon. It is possible to have a disease but not be distressed. Indeed, it is possible to be dying and not be distressed.

The body becomes an interface for the expression of identity that is personal and social. In a metaphysical tradition, the human being is considered as a self-contained consciousness, *homo clausus*; yet Smith (1999) argues for an alternative model, *homo aperti*, the idea that human beings gain identity through participation in social groups. My argument so far is that this identity is performed and that both personal and social are necessary; that the interaction of personal and social is circular and the difference between them constructed. Bodies express themselves at the interface of the personal and the social. Using the body communicates to others. Using the body achieves perception of the environment, which includes those with whom we live. The body has perhaps been neglected in communication studies as we emphasize language, yet it is gesture that is pre-verbal and promotes thought. Posture, movement and prosodics in relationship provide the bases for communication. Through the medium of an active performed body, health is expressed and maintained. Here is the bodily form that guides communication and by which the other may be understood and has an ambiguous content. It is social. Language provides a specific content. It is cultural. We know that someone is suffering by their appearance; what the specific nature of that suffering is they need to tell us. We know someone is happy by what they do; what makes them so happy they need to tell us. In addition, by moving as if we were happy, we may promote happiness. By moving as if we were sad, we may promote sadness. Thus the body, and a moved body at that, is central to a life among others.

Language is a means of performing an authored personal identity and this occurs through narratives that are located within a cultural context (Aldridge 1998). Narratives are not only related but are also heard. This is the social. Healing is concerned with offering social contexts for the expression of healing narratives. These social contexts are embodied in acts of 'being for the other' and entail the performance of shared meanings. This is the praxis aesthetic of health referred to in Chapter 4.

Making sense of adversity

Making sense of adversity is what we do when we are a patient. We connect our illnesses to a specific biography. We weave together events and episodes from daily life incorporating the bruises and kisses together into a life story: a potential life story, for once we enter into the healing narrative that story is subjected to various interpretations according to the company we keep. As we saw in the suicide book, the legitimation of those stories is crucial to the process of healing (Aldridge 1998). Thus while we will have self-authored identities, they are dependent upon dialogue.

Csordas (1983) writes that it is not the removal of symptoms that is important from a healing perspective, but an alteration in lifestyle and a change in the meaning of personal attributes related to illness. This is a meaning centred discussion rather than a disease centred discussion:

> Healing is treated as a discourse that activates and gives meaningful form to endogenous physiological and psychological healing processes in the patient. This discourse has three basic components: a rhetoric of disposition, a rhetoric of empowerment and a rhetoric of transformation. The net effect of therapy is to redirect the patient's attention to various aspects of his life in such a way as to create a new meaning for that life, and a transformed sense of himself as a whole and well person. (Csordas 1983, p.360).

Predisposition refers to an individual believing that healing is possible and the means of healing are legitimate. Empowerment is being persuaded that the therapy is efficacious and transformation is that change, however it may appear, is recognized.

An authored identity

Language is important for the way in which we author our identities and, as I shall go on to argue, if health is an important factor of identity, then the language options we have for 'authoring' ourselves are vital. The language of spirituality enhances the repertoires of healing vocabularies which we have by transforming and transcending understandings. A vocabulary that includes hope, transcendence, forgiveness and grace will be important in how we author our identity. In religious terms, ritual provides a means of authoring identity through action and involvement with a given vocabulary and grammar. George Orwell demonstrated the totalitarianism inherent in the destruction of words that makes 'the vocabulary smaller and the range of thoughts narrower' (Markova 1997). Including a spiritual vocabulary and the rituals in which it can be used offers us a greater variety of options for constructing identities. If we lose the opportunity to exercise the language of spirituality, or the religious contexts in which such language can be performed, then we are significantly impoverishing the healing cultures in which we live. More than that, with the loss of the language we lose the concepts involved. As we will see in Chapter 5, the retelling of lives, a performance in the company of others, invigorated by a spiritual understanding, brings about a transcendental change in health.

A performed identity

Yet, there is another profound level of understanding that lies beyond, or before, verbal communication. Underlying an authored identity is the notion that we 'do' who we are. We perform our very selves in the world as activities. This is a basic as our physiology and the grounds of immunology, a performance of the self to maintain its identity. Over and above this, we have the performance of a personality, not separate from the body, for which the body serves as an interface to the social world. We also perform that self among other performers. We have a social world in which we 'do' our lives with others. This is the social self that is recognized and acknowledged by our friends, lovers and colleagues. This performed identity is not solely dependent upon language, but it is composed rather like a piece of jazz. We are improvised each day to meet the contingencies of that day; and improvised with others, who may prove to be the very contingencies that day has to offer. We perform our identities and they have to have form for communication to occur. Such form is like musical form. Language provides the content for those per-form-ances. Thus we need an authored identity to express the distress in a coherent way with others to generate intelligible accounts (Csordas 1983). We have a network of coherent symbols.

Prayer, meditation and worship will not simply be expressive ways of communicating with others in the world about ourselves, they are also means of understanding the world through others. But those activities have to be per-formed and interpreted and are simply not cognitive activities alone. Prayer has its posture and movement too and through its posture we understand and demonstrate. We need both *form* and *meaning*. Similarly, public prayer has its liturgy. In the architecture of a liturgy we have a cultural understanding that is performed and transmitted. That is the performative purpose of ritual, it provides both form and meaning. Csordas describes this too as a creative opportunity for achieving 'the sacred self' (1997). As we will see in Chapter 3, Durkheim has already offered the idea that it is the social that provides form, as categories, by which the individual understands the world. It is culture that elaborates those categories as specific understandings through individual action. It is individual bodies that are the sites for the expression of the cultural in social relationship such that those sacred selves are realized.

Health identities are authored by individuals. There are, however, dangers in self-definitions of identity, as we will see in Chapter 4. We are open to an inherent narcissism. If this narcissism is combined with the omnipresence of globalized trivialities, then we reduce the alternatives of an actively lived healing repertoire still further. Furthermore, in the search for personal entitlements to health and in the struggle for the freedom of self-expression through self-fulfilment, then we are in danger of losing the social commitment that offers a transcending perspective. We may be free to fulfil ourselves according to our entitlements, but rarely do we consider that such fulfilment may be a loss or limitation if the offerings are impoverished or trivialized. Perhaps such egocentricity is a limited potential and there is more to us than what we know, as the great spiritual traditions would have us believe. To develop a consciousness for a broader potential is a goal of spiritual and religious teaching. Spiritual teachings have emphasized that we may achieve a higher self, a broadening of our current perspective, and this can be achieved through transformation. This transformation is facilitated by the relational contexts in which we have our daily lives.

Anecdotes

Complementary medical approaches are often dismissed as relying upon anecdotal material, as if stories are unreliable. My argument is that stories are reliable and rich in information. Indeed, it is a complaint made by patients of modern medical practitioners that they are not allowed to tell their own stories and a reason given why they turn to alternative medical practitioners who give them time to explain their problem in their own terms. While we as medical scientists may try and dismiss the anecdote, we rely upon it when we wish to explain particular cases to our colleagues away from the conference podium (Aldridge 1991b). Even in scientific medicine, it has been the single case report that has been necessary to alert practitioners to the negative side effects of current treatment.

While anecdotes may be considered as bad science, they are the everyday stuff of clinical practice. People tell us their stories and expect to be heard. Stories have a structure and are told in a style that informs us too. It is not solely the content of a story but how it is told that convinces us of its validity. While questionnaires gather information about populations and view the world from the perspective of the researcher, it is the interview which provides the condition for the patient to generate his meaningful story. The relationship is the context for the story and patients' stories may change according to the conditions in which they are related. This raises significant validity problems for questionnaire research. Anecdotes are the very stuff of social life and the fabric of communication in the healing encounter. As Miller (1998a) writes:

> Every time the experimental psychologist writes a research report in which anecdotal evidence has been assiduously avoided, the experimental scientist is generating anecdotal evidence for the consumption of his/her colleagues. (p.246)

The research report itself is an anecdotal report.

Stories play an important role in the healing process and that testimony is an important consideration. Indeed, we have to trust each other in what we say. This is the basis of human communication in the human endeavour of healing.

2

Meaning, purpose and power

The conservative laws of energy and matter are concerned with substance rather than form. Mental process, ideas, communication, organization, differentiation, pattern and so on, are matters of form rather than substance. (Gregory Bateson 1972)

When a man looks at the ocean he can only see that part of it which comes within his range of vision. So it is with the Truth. (Inayat Khan 1979)

Meaning and the ecology of mind

Throughout this book it will be emphasized that when studying human behaviour we must look at the context in which that behaviour is part and the closely related phenomenon of meaning. When we explain meaning, the act of interpretation, then we are mapping data onto events. When we observe we are concerned with the basic act of induction. Yet these observations must be fitted within a framework. This is referred to earlier as an ecology of ideas. But, as we saw in Chapter 1, this is not solely about ideas and beliefs, emotions or cognitions, it is about how those ideas are acted upon; not simply the interpretation of meaning but the consequences of acting upon meanings.

In a previous book about suicide (Aldridge 1998), the interpretation of meaning is understood as being based upon constitutive rules that lend events coherence. Yet these rules of meaning alone are not enough. There is another set of related rules that determined the consequences of understanding, that is, regulative rules. Understanding how a person interprets the meaning of an event is one thing, but what they do about it is something else. While we need to know what events mean, we also need to know what to do.

Constitutive rules and regulative rules are nested as a hierarchy of understandings. Individuals interpret the world in a particular way and these interpretations are based upon a relational set of rules that in turn are based upon cultural rules. In this way, a man in his forties who has committed a crime and is facing prosecution becomes depressed, sees his life as having no further meaning and decides that it is legitimate to kill himself. His wife, however, may see that this is a temporary state of distress and can be reconciled. For her, their marriage is a reason for him to go on living and so his suicide is illegitimate. At a societal level, he is considered deviant, potentially criminal, appropriately distressed and, considering his age, his suicide is legitimate.

These aspects of rule-governed behaviour and the interpretation of meaning, when applied to understanding a person's life and its purpose within social contexts and informed culturally, are hallmarks of varying definitions of spirituality and religion, as we will see later in this chapter (see Reese 1997 in Table 2.5). However, it is important to see that these rules are local and temporary. These are not laws as in a natural scientific sense, nor are they laws as in a legal sense. They are not fixed or immutable. Thinking and behaviour follow patterns. Those patterns are discernible. Those discernible patterns appear to follow rules, but these rules are flexible and multilayered. Sometimes these rules appear as codes of conduct and commandments when religions attempt to stabilize a particular social grouping.

The pattern that connects

The concept of an ecology of ideas is taken from the work of Gregory Bateson (1972, 1978, 1991) and I shall come back to his work several times throughout this book. Bateson's thesis is that there are patterns which can be identified in human behaviour. In the idea of an ecology, where there are interconnecting patterns, there is a meta-pattern that connects. Discovering the meta-pattern that connects is the discovery of the sacred. For Bateson it is the relation of the microcosm of the human being as it reflects and partakes of the macrocosm of nature. This connection I shall refer to as a horizontal ecology connecting systems within material and organizational constellations. However, what is necessary to take from Bateson is his insistence that there is a pattern which connects and that we recognize such patterns. While the components of a pattern on a tiled floor, for example, are the tiles, the pattern itself is the way in which they are arranged. This pattern, as arrangement, is non-material. Throughout this book I shall be referring to material events and how they appear in sickness. What is important is to consider how those events are interpreted as patterns of illness and then classified as to their meanings and causes. This is a process of recognition as re-cognition. As re-search, in research, is looking again to discover the new, re-cognition is thinking again to discover the pattern that connects. Thus recognition of a connecting pattern is the basis of knowledge.

Table 2.1 Spirituality, meaning and unity

Spirit refers to that noncorporeal and nonmental dimension of the person that is the source of unity and meaning, and 'spirituality' refers to the concepts, attitudes, and behaviours that derive from one's experience of that dimension. Spirit can be addressed only indirectly and inferentially, while spirituality can be understood and worked with in psychologic terms. (p.742)	(Hiatt 1986)
Not only of belief in God but of a relationship with a supreme power, often a relationship that includes prayer in some form. Others speak of the conviction that life has a purpose, of the search from meaning, of the attempt to interpret their present illness in a way that makes sense within their world-view. (p.87)	(Smyth and Bellemare 1988)
Spiritual…means in essence 'searching for existential meaning'. Spiritual beliefs may be expressed in religion and its hallowed practices, but a person can and often does have a spiritual dimension to his or her life that is totally unrelated to religion and not expressed or explored in religious practice. (p.303)	(Doyle 1992)
Definitions of spirituality…referred to a dynamic, principle, or an aspect of a person that related to God or god, other persons, or aspects of personal being or material nature… The spiritual dimension was used to refer to a quality beyond religious affiliation that is used to inspire or harmonize answers to questions regarding infinite subjects, e.g., meaning and purpose of life and one's relation to the universe. (p.43)	(Emblen 1992)
It is useful to think of spirit, spirituality, and religion as different points on a continuum. Spirit is the source dimension behind every personal or collective experience of spirituality. It is also the source dimension behind every religion. Spirituality can be considered closer to the source dimension than everyday religion that has moved far from the experience of spirit and primarily serves moral and social purposes. Spirit is said…to be the realm that unites us. (p.115)	(Lerner 1994)
(a) the need to find meaning, purpose and fulfilment in life, suffering and death, (b) the need for hope/will to live, (c) the need for belief and faith in self, others and God. (p.439)	(Ross 1994)
Spirituality is…the experiential integration of one's life in terms of one's ultimate values and meanings. (p.330)	(Muldoon and King 1995)
A quality that goes beyond religious affiliation, that strives for inspirations, reverence, awe and purpose…tries to be in harmony with the universe, strives for answers about the infinite, and comes into focus when the person faces emotional stress, physical illness or death. (p.413)	(McSherry and Draper 1997)
Spirituality is a belief system focusing on intangible elements that impart vitality and meaning to life events. (p.220)	(Joseph 1998)

Table 2.2 Spirituality as transcendental	
Spirituality is defined in terms of personal views and behaviors that express a sense of relatedness to a transcendent dimension or to something greater than the self... Spirituality is a broader concept than religion or religiosity ... Indicators of spirituality include prayer, sense of meaning in life, reading and contemplation, sense of closeness to a higher being, interactions with others and other experiences which reflect spiritual interaction or awareness. Spirituality may vary according to developmental level and life events. (p.336)	(Reed 1987)
Spiritual elements are those capacities that enable a human being to rise above or transcend any experience at hand. They are characterized by the capacity to seek meaning and purpose, to have faith, to love, to forgive, to pray, to meditate, to worship, and to seek beyond present circumstances. (p.91)	(Kuhn 1988)
The spiritual dimension of persons can be uniquely defined as the human capacity to transcend self, which is phenomenologically reflected in three basic spiritual needs: (a) the need for self-acceptance, a trusting relationship with self based on a sense of meaning and purpose in life; (b) the need for relationship with others and/or a supreme other (e.g. God) characterized by nonconditional love, trust, and forgiveness; and (c) the need for hope, which is the need to imagine and participate in the enhancement of a positive future. All persons experience these spiritual needs, whether or not they are part of a formal religious organization. (p.3)	(Highfield 1992)
Spiritual: pertaining to the innate capacity to, and tendency to seek to, transcend one's current locus of centricity, which transcendence involves increased love and knowledge. (p.169)	(Chandler, Holden and Kolander 1992)
Six clear factors...appear to be fundamental aspects of spirituality ... those of the journey, transcendence, community, religion, 'the mystery of creation,' and transformation. (p.154)	(Lapierre 1994)
Spirituality...pertains to one's relationship with others, with oneself and with one's higher power, which is defined by the individual and need not be associated with a formal religion. (p.287)	(Borman and Dixon 1998)
Spirituality refers to the degree of involvement or state of awareness or devotion to a higher being or life philosophy. Not always related to conventional beliefs. (p.65)	(Lukoff *et al.* 1999)
Spirituality is rooted in an awareness which is part of the biological make-up of the human species. Spirituality is present in all individuals and it may manifest as inner peace and strength derived from perceived relationship with a transcendent God or an ultimate reality or whatever an individual values as supreme. (p.124)	(Narayana-samy 1999)

Yet, there is also a vertical relationship which all major religions recognize as a spiritual dimension and that is the relationship between the human being and the divine. We see this reflected in the Yin and Yang symbol of traditional Chinese medicine that emphasizes the vertical relationship between the human and the divine, each in their manifestation containing a seed of the other and uniting together to form a whole. Similarly, the Christian cross reflects both the realms of horizontal earthly existence and vertical divine relationship. The difficulty lies in the explanations that are used for understanding when either a sacred ecology or the divine relationship is used. One is assumed to supersede the other according to the interpreter of events. Both are partial. Indeed, what many spiritual authors seek is to take us beyond the dualisms of material and spiritual, beyond body and mind, to realize that in understanding the relations between the two then we leap to another realm of knowledge. Indeed, the Buddhist concept of the 'Middle Way' is not to find some mid-point between the two, but to transcend the two ideas unifying them in a balanced understanding. Postmodern understandings would want to remove these very concepts of 'Divine' and science as grand narratives, taking away the very notion that there is a universal. All that we have is what there is before us and even this is what we have constructed ourselves. I shall not be taking such a radical constructivist stance in this book and the arguments may perhaps be better expressed as late modern. I am assuming an absolute truth with a plurality of perspectives on that truth that we find in the varying sciences, art, philosophy and religion.

Science and religion as ways of knowing

While it is necessary to speak of matter and, I argue here, also of spirit, the use of those words tends to separate. This is in the nature of language. We merely have to be aware that we are separating understandings. The diamond cutter uses such knowledge to cleave the stone and present it in its best light by varying the facets; so too with our knowledge of what it is to be human. We present the varying facets as they lend their brilliance to the way in which we choose to present the stone of knowledge. One of these facets is that of natural science, but there are others which are also of interest. To extend this metaphor further, culture would be the setting that is fashioned to hold the stone of science in all its brilliance. However, the jewel that is art could be just as easily substituted. Both may be admired for their clarity or beauty, but it is the setting that enables them achieve their function; so too with religion.

The word science in its English usage springs from the Latin *scire*, to know, originally meaning to cut and thereby to decide, and has a relationship with the Latin adjective *scius*, meaning 'knowing'. So, on the one hand we have a derivation of science that appears to be about making decisions, to cut and to separate, as we saw in the previous metaphor of the diamond cutter and the stone for knowledge.

Or, we can follow another route and look at the adjective *scius* as it refers to knowing and as it occurs in the Latin word *conscius*, literally con = together, scius = knowing). Perhaps this is what we are searching for in our scientific activity – how we can share knowledge or how we can bring knowledge into consciousness. Bringing knowledge into consciousness is the basis of spirituality. Bringing a scientific understanding and an existential understanding, heart and intellect, together is an act of consciousness. If science contains the first notion of decision or judgement, doing science – or the activity of sciencing – is a matter of deciding. It is therefore also an ethical activity.

Yet another element of science stems from its root in *sapientia*, as vision. Vision in this sense is a way of looking at the world and the way that the world looks at us. From this perspective, we have world views and comparative visions that may be scientific, theological, anthropological or aesthetic. While visionary may be applied to spiritual teachers, it has also surely been applied to those scientists in search of quarks and bacilli.

If we return to the roots of the everyday words which we use in medicine, then we see that spiritual considerations are not strange. Patient is derived from the Latin *pati*, which is to suffer and patiently endure. Doctor is the teacher who discerns from the Latin *docilitas*. Therapy is attentive support from the Greek *therapeutikos*. Therapist and doctor accompany the patient in their suffering along the way, with the responsibility of the healer to reach out to the patient and the doctor to discern and teach. Such a stance is not solely concerned with cure. There are also the possibilities of relief from suffering and comfort for the sick. Discernment is a broad term and includes not only the technical abilities of reading test results, but also implies an ability to understand the psychological and social needs of the patient. To this we can add further dimension and that is to discern the spiritual needs of a patient. When a person's suffering is related to a question asking why they have been abandoned, then they are reflecting the central question of Christianity, of Christ upon the cross asking his god why he has been abandoned. When a patient asks, 'If I had treated my wife a little better over the years would this maybe not have happened to her?', then we are hearing a psychological difficulty related to guilt but also reflecting a need for forgiveness. While one spouse may be sick, the other suffers also. Forgiveness is considered in this book as a spiritual dimension in Chapter 6 and is seen as an important variable in relieving suffering.

Spirituality and religion in medicine

While medicine indeed may try to look like a natural science and is sometimes scientific, in its practice and delivery it is not (Moerman 1998). Medical practice exists as the humane action of one human being toward another to provide comfort, relief and sometimes to cure (van Leeuwen and Kimsma 1997). Fabrega

(1997, p.26) writes succinctly that: 'If disease, injury and physiological processes are the biologically based substrates of the medical, then sickness (the socially constructed expression of a subjective state of illness) and healing (the socially constructed efforts, procedures, and medicines aimed at neutralising illness) are its social and cultural realizations.' I would argue that spirituality too is a substrate worth considering in the health-care discourse.

How we understand healing in medicine will be influenced by the philosophy of science that we have. My proposal is that science is a process, an activity not a set of commandments set in stone for all time as the basis for a dogma. Science does not have to conform to one particular perspective on the world. There are varying sciences of geography, meteorology and agriculture that we consider important within a modern culture for constructing knowledge. But these sciences do not mean that in other generations other peoples could not find their way from one region to another, predict the weather or grow crops successfully. This is not an argument for discarding the sciences, simply for recognizing the place of the sciences, the partiality of explicit knowledge and the pragmatic value of experiential knowledge.

Yet another perspective would take us to the German word for science, *Wissenschaft*. *Wissen* is to know or to know about and is related to knowledge and judgement, while *schaffen* is to make or create, to manage or accomplish. So, from another European perspective, we see science as an activity of creating knowledge as a form of judgement. Perhaps it is this creative activity that may appeal to many of us today and that some of us feel has become lost to the scientific activity. Knowledge is something that can be done; it is a creative activity, a process, not a fixed product. Indeed the word knowledge in English is distantly derived from a root that means 'I can' (Middle English as Ic can and in German as *können* and *kennen*) and is best described as the statement 'I can know'. Once we take such a position of knowledge being actively acquired, then we can speculate upon the various arts of doing science. The basis of the scientific activity will be in the presentation of forms of knowledge, some of which will be empirically based. From a spiritual perspective, it is the gaining of this knowledge that is important and this will have a variety of sources. In my book on music therapy (Aldridge 1996) I have argued that through the creative arts we have an alternative view of human beings, as created works of art not mechanical structures, and that knowledge of the world is gained as an aesthetic expressive activity. In the following literature related to spirituality in healing contexts we will also see how people gain knowledge of themselves through the experience of illness and suffering.

How do we create knowledge, then? This question lies at the centre of many modern scientific debates and is a question of methodology. One of our critiques of modern science is that the argument rarely concentrates on the subject matter of our inquiry which leads to a new creative discovery for the person who wants to know. The activity of science seems more like the pressure for us to conform in our knowing to a set of prescriptions which are applied to a given body of knowledge, that is, methodolatry not methodology. It is this struggle with an appropriate methodology that we find in the current healing literature and one that has been hotly debated during the last decade within the field of complementary medicine. What I am trying to do here is to argue for a plurality of knowledge. Plurality assumes that there is an absolute truth but because of our human limitations we, not being divine or supreme beings, can only have bounded understandings. Our challenge then is to begin to understand how those bounded understandings fit together; to recognize the pattern that connects; to transcend our limitations in what we know.

An historical perspective

Medicine has a system of explanations for what it does. These are claimed to be predominantly scientific and it was a coherence of cogent ideas that was influential historically in the separation of scientific medicine from the influence of the church and metaphysical notions of healing. The history of the spiritual in healing throughout varying epochs reflects the growth of scientific knowledge, demands for religious renewal and the continuing shift of understanding concerning what is health within a broader cultural context.

Historically, ideas regarding healing fell into two main schools: ritualistic healing, whereby people fall ill and are restored to health through psychic or spiritual forces; and mechanistic healing, whereby people become ill following over-indulgence, sitting in damp places or changes in the weather and are restored by purges, diet and the unblocking of energies. These schools are not mutually exclusive and the idea of healing energies is common to both, uniting them in forms of treatment while separating them in terms of diagnostics according to causative forces and causative materials.

The sacred disease 'epilepsy', which included hysteria and demonic possession, believed to be caused by the entry of the gods into mortal bodies to serve divine purposes, came to be challenged in the fifth century (Inglis 1979) as the invocation of divine elements masked the inability to provide effective treatment. With the questioning of spiritual causation, then material causes were sought, the consequence of which was the theory of the 'four humours' which must be balanced to maintain the status of health within the body. These theories eventually led to modern physiology and allopathic remedies.

Throughout the last two thousand years Christian healing, reviving vitalist theories and shifting away from Greek concepts of hygiene, survived under the threat of Roman persecution by inspiring followers through acts of healing and other inspirational gifts. Christ's injunction to his disciples was to heal the sick.

The restoration of faith through acts of repentance and the sacrament of healing could restore the person to health. In these early accounts body and soul were not separate. A soul restored to holiness (wholeness) – the root word of health and healing – was also a healthy body. In these terms wholeness means a return to unity with God and is achieved by the action of the spirit.

What is important in this early Christian tradition, and particularly for the miracles worked by Jesus, is that these healing miracles, along with the others, were examples of spiritual transformations intended to initiate the receiver. The process of healing was instrumental to reunite the person with the divine. In several instances, the person being healed is instructed not to tell others about what has happened. If we take this example literally, from a fundamentalist perspective, then we could not use case studies of spiritual healing to tell others when such a healing takes place. Shah (1990) writes that this concealment is to prevent an over-emotionalization of such events that publicity and excitement brings and to prevent the slide into superstition. All too often, Jesus is identified as a prototypical nurse or doctor rather than the spiritual teacher whom he was. Little wonder then that spiritual healing is often judged in terms of modern health-care demands of objective outcomes and symptom relief. Such outcomes are seen as shallow emotional expectations of a higher understanding, albeit medically appropriate.

Healing as a restoration of souls in their unity with God became an important element in the early evangelical endeavour. Such an ecological understanding is not far from modern (w)holistic understandings. However, with the removal of God from the postmodern debate then we have potentially removed that wholeness to which we can aspire. While this vision may have been supplanted by the functional productive body as the subject of modern medicine, it has perhaps proved to be unsatisfactory for its users searching for something more sublime.

As Christianity gradually became accepted and established, healing, which depended upon individuals being inspired by the spirit as opposed to being licensed by law, was seen as a threat to the hierarchy of the church. Eventually, in the twelfth century, Pope Alexander was to ban spiritual healing as a suspect activity, inspired by the devil to seduce unwitting clergy to deal with matters of the flesh and all its temptations. Such material concerns were best left to physicians.

Furthermore, the physicians began to organize themselves into guilds and medicine began to form itself into a body of knowledge replicable in university centres throughout Europe. Metaphysics became increasingly idiosyncratic and open to individual interpretation and sentimentality. Christianity surrendered the sole authority to speak of life, birth and death to a materialistic science that verified human life in the same way in which it verified the physical universe (Needleman 1988). Understandings of the body and its relation to illness were transformed in the seventeenth century by the ability to dissect corpses (Foucault 1989). Observation of externals gave way to the examination of internals, which in itself led to a different classification for disease. Supernatural explanations and causative forces were rejected in favour of theories about living bodies within the realm of material phenomena, albeit discovered from corpses. Similarly academic medicine in the universities became separated from the empirical practice of clinicians observing the effects of their ministrations. That the human body could be organized by subtle forces and represented the presence of a higher intelligence in the universe was abandoned (Hossein Nasr 1990). Thus we see a rift in the ecology of ideas. The material becomes separated from those subtle influences that play upon it and of which it is part. Priests minister the soul, a soul that is evermore separated from spirit, and physicians attend the body. However, within recent times we have seen a return to the idea that body, mind and spirit are not separate.

Meanings

'If you want to find satisfactory formulas you had better deal with things that can be fitted into a formula. The vocation to seek God is not one of them. Nor is existence. Nor is the spirit of man' (Merton 1996, p.138).

Hiatt (1986), as a psychiatrist, offers an understanding of the spiritual in medicine which can be worked with in psychologic terms:

Spirit refers to that noncorporeal and nonmental dimension of the person that is the source of unity and meaning, and 'spirituality' refers to the concepts, attitudes, and behaviours that derive from one's experience of that dimension. Spirit can be addressed only indirectly and inferentially, while spirituality can be understood and worked with in psychologic terms. (Hiatt 1986, p.742)

He suggests that by taking such a psychologic framework then we can discuss and use spiritual healing 'within a modified western framework (of medicine)' (p.742; see Table 2.1). Lerner has taken this definition one step further and offers a pragmatic understanding of spirituality and religion where spirit is inferred as an implicate unifying force that is explicated in various religious practices. In this way, we would see differing social groups in varying cultures being informed by spirit but realizing quite different forms of ritual, worship and religious practice.

Spirituality in a late modern sense is used consistently throughout the literature related to medical practice as an ineffable dimension that is separate from religion itself. A person may regard herself as having a spiritual dimension, but this may not be explored in any religious practice. Similarly she may be involved in religious practices but without any spiritual dimension (Doyle 1992; Emblen 1992).

Central to these arguments is the concept that spirituality lends a unity and purpose to life (Doyle 1992; Emblen 1992; McSherry and Draper 1997; Ross 1994). Psychiatry has made an effort within the last decade to include spirituality and bases its definitions primarily on the idea of a force or power that informs belief, promotes meaning and purpose or maintains motivation (King and Dein 1998; King, Speck and Thomas 1995a; Sims 1994). Writers in psychological medicine have attempted to gather the relevant literature together and discuss a suitable definition relevant for clinical practice (Lukoff, Lu and Turner 1998; Lukoff *et al.* 1999). It is often expressed that in palliative care, the existential meaning of life gains importance during the process of dying and this reflects a spiritual dimension (Doyle 1992; Ross 1995). McSherry and Draper (1997) emphasize a unifying aspect of spirituality that tries to bring the person in harmony with the universe and offer answers about the infinite, a dimension that comes to the fore when a person is ill or faces death. What some of us may also argue is that meaning and purpose are vital throughout life, not only during the dying process, and when lost result in hopelessness and despair (Aldridge 1998).

Suffering as loss of unity

Illness, from this perspective of spiritual meaning, occurs when unity is lost and a person becomes separated from the ground of her being. She becomes a refugee within her own soul. The outbreak of illness indicates a seeking of the self to attract attention to factors that are preventing a realization of unity. In the process of attempted suicide, we see how some people are not trying to kill themselves but indeed to heal a relational system that is falling apart either by stimulating change or by slowing down changes that seem to be happening too quickly. Attempted suicide is a way of saying 'something is dying if change does not happen'. Rather than simply a negative activity, the process may be a way of stimulating healing to occur, albeit drastically. The same argument applies to chronic illness. It is an attempt to promote healing by bringing attention through suffering to changes that need to occur. From a spiritual perspective both the suffering and the nature of the illness have value, to restore a condition of wholeness – as health – and as a teaching vehicle. We learn about ourselves through suffering. Even when an illness does not disappear, we can cope and live lives in fullness. This has led some authors to propose coping strategies related to spiritual well-being (Ganzevoort 1998), particularly in the elderly (Chang, Noonan and Tennstedt 1998; Clark *et al.* 1996; Krause 1998), those suffering with cancer (Carr and Morris 1996; Irving, Snyder and Crowson 1998) and after surgery (Tix and Frazier 1998).

I am not advocating that we embrace suffering for its own sake. Indeed, the teaching dimension here is supplementary to that of healing the illness. But, there is an heuristic value here for understanding chronic illness. Through the process of understanding what the illness means for the patient and his family, then we may achieve some longer term healing. Our lives and how we live them with those we love may need to change. This argument is not far removed from the principles of family therapy where illness is seen in its systemic context. If we consider chronic heart disease, where there has to be an immediate physical intervention, it is only by understanding the long-term psychological needs of the patient and his family situation that compliance with medical treatment will be achieved. If that very same person is suffering spiritually, doubting what purpose his life has, then these medical, psychological and social interventions will be seriously undermined. Decisions about wanting to live will be paramount and need to be addressed. This is not an argument to abandon the medical, rather that we contextualize our clinical medical interventions within an appropriate framework of understanding: in this instance, the spiritual.

Healing arises from within the patient as a search for wholeness. This wholeness refers not just to a necessary physical integrity but also to the connection with a broader unity. Without a sense of purpose, life's intent, then we have nothing.

The restoration of unity

Those practitioners writing about spirituality emphasize its multiple dimensions (see Table 2.1). Most of them present some sort of force that may not directly be perceived, but of which we are aware and which lends vitality to the meaning of life events (Hiatt 1986; Joseph 1998) that itself leads to a sense of an ultimate reality which brings a significance and sense of purpose to what we do. This reality is said to be beyond the senses, the physical world being only one perceptive reality that is available to us. It is ineffable and totally subjective, making itself elusive to scientific inquiry. It is an experiential activity, not an aspect of thought, and is in a constant state of dynamic flux. When these experiences emerge as thoughts, or as states of energy, then they become amenable to description and it is here that we may begin to investigate them in terms of behavioural and psychological medicine.

The danger is that some of these behaviours, like the pursuance of ecstatic states or the achievement of trance, may become dislocated from their spiritual intentions. Thus we may be tempted to secularize the practice for its physiological benefits divorced from an understanding of the spiritual source. To do so is to remove the central integrative plank of the spirituality argument which is that of restoring unity to a fragmented experiential world providing both direction and harmony. This unity provides a context for living. The psychological value will be in concrete understandings as they provide direction and the physical dimension will be the energy available for putting understandings into practice. For those who have worked with patients who are chronically depressed, then it is the process of thinking that needs to be changed and accommodated within a broader life perspective combined with the necessary energy to act. If the source of depression is that the person finds no meaning or purpose in this life, then a spiritual awakening will have important ramifications for his recovery. For the alcoholic, as we will see in Chapter 5, this change of thought and action which follows a spiritual awakening is the key to recovery (Borman and Dixon 1998; Kurtz 1979). It is not simply the change in thinking that has to occur, but the necessary actions have to take place. It is here that religion has previously offered the appropriate stages to combine the two, as we will read later.

Spirituality, then, is considered to be a force or power bringing about ineffable experiences that promote purpose and unity. These may be unrelated to religious beliefs and worship practices (Emblen 1992). The result of this power is often to promote transcendence either from the material realm or from the current situation.

Beyond meaning

Medicine, from the Latin root *medicus*, is the measure of illness and injury, and shares the Latin *metiri*, to measure. Yet this measurement was based on natural cycles and measures. To attend medically, Latin *mederi*, also supports the Latin word *meditari* from which we have the modern meditation, which is the measuring of an idea in thought. The task of the healer in this sense is to direct the attention of the patient through the value of suffering to a solution which is beyond the problem itself. In this sense, the healer encourages a change in the sign of the patient's suffering from negative to positive. We are encouraged to see the benefit of suffering in bringing us beyond our present understandings, which is also an understanding of the transcendental.

In Table 2.2 we see how a variety of writers have tackled this perspective of transcendence in emphasizing 'going beyond' a current awareness to another level of understanding. This does not necessarily imply a conventional set of beliefs. It is based upon an innate capacity that we have as human beings to rise above the situation. While this appears to be a personal constructivist argument based on an innate capacity, it assumes that there is also an Other, either as a higher being or as partner greater than the self. It is at this point where Boyd (1995) makes his argument for a consideration of the term 'soul' as separate from 'spirit'. 'Soul' is the subjective or inner person as a whole in the natural state, including the body as an inseparable part, and relates to the word 'psyche' (p.151). 'Spirit' however refers to that which could be both inside and outside a person. Soul focuses on the secular self; spirit refers to that which brings the soul to transcend itself, from without or within.

Chandler, Holden and Kolander (1992) see the search for meaning as a central process for the human being related to 'questioning'. Indeed, the process of spiritual development is seen as a 'quest' or journey. In medieval times the quest for the Holy Grail was not for a material chalice but symbolized the search for knowledge as a vessel in which the divine may be contained. However, what confounds this issue today is that we equate questioning as an activity rather like the chatter of infants. Many spiritual traditions emphasize the importance of silence and non-activity where the appropriate question may be framed and, as importantly, the answer may be heard. Meditation and prayer have both been used to fulfil these functions. As we shall read later, the difficulty is that prayer is usurped actively to seek material benefits and loses its contemplative nature and the opportunity to discern answers.

Techniques of questioning, as embarking upon a quest, are at the heart of both science and spirituality in the search for knowledge. However, both demand a discipline if answers are to be found. These appropriate methods of questioning have to be learned and the approaches taught. The answers however cannot be learned for they appear new to each generation and to the appropriate contexts.

Transcendence

As a process, transcendence is seen as taking us beyond our small selves, outside the everyday limitations of personality. In a step beyond egocentricty, rejecting narcissism, we take an enlightened interest in others and the world through which we are led to a greater knowledge and a capacity to love. This may mean moving away from former friends and family as reference points. Again, in conversations with suicidal patients and their families, it was this search by adolescents and young adults for a newer fulfilling life that brought them away from those former reference points. An existential demand for change brought about uncertainty, even when it was necessary. It appeared that something was dying. And if something was dying, the way that things were had to die, thus the metaphor of attempted suicide. In the spiritual traditions we see the same metaphor, that we must die before we can live. That is not to say that there has to be a literal death, simply that the old self must be discarded to be reborn to a new self.

At such moments of change, where new identities emerge, then counselling is appropriate. Most spiritual traditions and secular approaches have developed techniques to enable that questioning to occur safely. If transcendence is the outcome of spiritual development, a development that is necessary for a life to unfold, then that development needs to be guided. Religious practices have provided this framework for achieving spiritual awareness within a cultural framework. These practices are based upon stages, from the novice to the enlightened, and the seeker is guided to discover her own understanding. Once religions become dogmatic practices and lose the understanding of stages, then they become inappropriate to the spiritual search. This appears to be the source of the rejection of traditional religious frameworks although spiritual needs remain as strong. Just as a teacher will gradually introduce a student to different realms of thinking and discovery in science, tailoring the teaching to adapt to the capacity of the student and his stages of development, then so it is with spiritual understanding.

Once religions begin to give answers and promote the dogma that 'God said' then they lose their spiritual vitality. Their task is to promote the abilities to question in the questioner and allow her to discover her own answer. Anything less than a trust in this process undermines the religion itself as it demonstrates a lack of trust in the sacred and promotes a secular authority.

Hard questions

'Why me? What did I do wrong? Haven't I tried to live my life in a proper way?' were questions that my friend George asked when he was diagnosed with leukaemia. And his wife asked me, 'Was it because we argued a lot last year? Would it have been different if I had treated him better?' Such questions occur when we work with those people and their families who are under the shadow of a life-threatening illness. It is not only the future that becomes uncertain, with questions about prognosis – the ubiquitous 'How long?' – but the past also comes into question. Identities are challenged. The self has to adapt to a new identity, albeit an identity under siege from a potential stigma; so do the identities of those with whom we live. How we transcend this situation and achieve a new identity has been described within the cancer nursing literature (Highfield 1992). Three basic needs are identified: a need for self-acceptance; a need for relationship with others, in particular a supreme other; and the need for hope. These needs are spiritual and not dependent upon participating in a religious organization.

Access to a higher power

While the spiritual dimension may be separate from the religious, religious practices are said to provide a bridge to the spiritual, thus assuming that the spiritual is a realm beyond the religious (Lukoff et al. 1999). This spiritual dimension is seen as a relationship with a higher power experienced as internal and intensely personal that need not be associated with the formal, external aspects of religion (Borman and Dixon 1998); transcending sense phenomena, rationality and feelings leading to a heightened state of consciousness or awareness (Lapierre 1994). The danger is that what may be seen as 'spiritual illuminations' in the raw condition of altered states of consciousness are imagined to be spiritual experiences. These can become addictive (Shah 1983, 1990) preventing any developmental change: thus the need for a spiritual guide, emphasized in the great traditions and reflected too in secular psychotherapy as a wise counsellor, to prevent the interpretation of emotions as spirituality.

When we come to examine the evidence of spiritual healing in the modern world then we must bear these considerations of purpose and transcendence in mind. The ability to rise above suffering, to go beyond the present situation to a realm where life takes on another perhaps deeper significance, is an important factor in palliative care, in the long-term management of chronic illness and as central plank of psychotherapy. In the treatment of alcoholism, it is the recognition of personal suffering and the need to transcend the limitations of the self, to understand that we are 'Not-God' (Kurtz 1979), as a process of spiritual awakening that brings about one of the vital steps in recovery.

Transcending the current situation

From the literature it is possible to piece together a process of spiritual change where there is a need to transcend the current situation. To achieve this there has to be a change both in thought and feeling accompanied by appropriate actions. This is expressed as a process of questioning, as a search for meaning. Such meanings take the searcher beyond what she is to a higher consciousness or state of awareness that is connected to the truth, which people refer to as 'god', 'the divine', 'the supreme power', 'that'. This is a circular process of development based on revealed personal understandings achieved through transcendence, which lead to other understandings. Idries Shah refers to this process as a removal of veils to the Truth (Shah 1978). These veils that obscure the truth are formed either through indoctrination, which blinds us, or through the base aspirations of our subjective selves preventing subtle perceptions and higher visions. Religion itself may be a veil that hides the truth, although it offers a public perspective into the truth (Gillespie 1998). The task we face is how to make those veils transparent or remove them. A further task is how to cope with the truth thus revealed.

Central to this process of transcendence is the recognition of a higher power. The argument surrounding powers, forces and energies appears to be a common denominator in varying explanations of spiritual healing. Even where spiritual energies are not mentioned directly in terms of healing, they are described as the driving force behind the specific search for meaning (Boyd 1995; King and Dein 1998) (see Table 2.3). So when we want to understand the process of healing, then perhaps we can use a coarse metaphor and ask how this process is fuelled. As we saw earlier, the whole person as 'soul' is transformed from within or without by 'spirit'. Perhaps commentators that refer to 'mind–body' medicine (Goleman and Gurin 1993) may be more accurate in referring to 'soul' medicine leaving room for an invigorated concept of spiritual healing.

Table 2.3 Spirituality as power or force	
There are numerous meanings for the word spiritual; the most useful imply what a person lives for, their motivating force; the weakest, a nebulous power beyond description. Here are five aspects of meaning which the psychiatrist should consider: ... looking for the meaning in life ... the interrelatedness of all ... wholeness of the person, in which spirit is not separate from body or mind ... what is seen as good, beautiful and enjoyable ... the connection between god and man. (p.444)	(Sims 1994)
We propose a definition of 'spiritual' as a person's experience of, or a belief in, a power apart from their own existence. It may exist within them but is ultimately apart. It is the sense of relationship or connection with a power or force. It is more specific than a search for meaning or unity with others. (p.1259)	(King and Dein 1998)
The spirit refers to what is inside a person; what we would call thoughts, feelings, energy, spirituality, the subjective viewpoint, mind, personality, psychology, or breath. But the spirit could also be outside a living person, and the implication would be that the internal spirit probably originated outside and invaded, so the person was 'inspired'. (p.155)	(Boyd 1995)

Vital energy

Explanations given for how such spiritual healing works are various: para-physical, magnetic, psychological and social. The prime explanatory principle is that there are divine energies which are transformed from the spiritual level by the agency of the healer and which produce a beneficial influence upon the 'energy field' of the patient.

In the 1920s there was an upsurge of interest in spirituality and spiritual healing following World War I and many of the descriptions used at that time were based on explanations of vibration (Khan 1974) where matter and spirit were seen as different manifestations of life. Matter is seen as a passing state of spirit: spirit being the organizing power, sometimes described metaphorically as 'magnetic power' or intelligence that brings the physical together. In modern terms we would translate this intelligence argument into one that talks of energy becoming organized by information. Some authors will describe organization as another form of energy. Thus modern energetic descriptions reflect traditional descriptions based on vibration, where there are levels of subtle vibrations experienced as the soul, denser vibrations experienced as feelings, yet denser vibrations of the material as seen in the body. Even that which is dead can be seen as material which vibrates, albeit slowly. My schoolboy understanding of atomic theory was also conveyed to me in such terms, that the molecular structure contained a vibratory world of seething atoms in varying states of excitation. How these atoms become organized as molecular structure or channelled into energy demands another order of description based on a concept of organization.

This notion of 'energy field' is the sticking point between orthodox researchers (Jacobs 1989; Wood 1989) and spiritual practitioners in that, if such a field exists, then it should be possible to measure by physical means. The problem probably lies in use of the word 'energy' that has a broader interpretation in spiritual healing and is likened to organizing principles of vitalism and life force which bring about a harmonizing of the whole person. The source of the word energy in the Greek is *ergon*, meaning both to work in a physical sense and to be active or possessed by a demon. The former is the meaning used by modern scientists; the latter by healers. If we add the prefix *en*, then we have *energio* – to be in action. In this sense it is used by modern spiritual healers to suggest dynamic forces that are channelled or set in motion by the healer, or the patient. Therefore, the energy of spirituality is the driving force that brings about transcendence, going beyond the current situation to that of wholeness.

Ancient systems of healing were based on the dynamic notion of energy (Leskowitz 1992). Fire energy brings warmth through the principle of motion. Hidden energy, which is air, is the sustaining energy and the activator of fire energy that uses the blood stream as its vehicle, thereby maintaining the chemistry of life and conveying the vital energies of the body. In addition, there are three forms of energy distribution: through the seven energy centres which serve as points of reception and distribution throughout the physical body; through the seven major glands of the endocrine system; and through the nervous system. Restriction or inhibition of the free flow of these energies creates an imbalance or disharmony in the others. Health can be restored by releasing the cause of the blockages and through the application of specific musical tones to restore the flow of energy.

While Sims (1994) (see Table 2.3) regards power descriptions as nebulous, other authors emphasize a power that may be internal or external to the person (King and Dein 1998; King *et al.* 1995a), the belief in which is more specific than a search for meaning (Boyd 1995). In the alcohol treatment literature, it is this belief in a higher power, as opposed to personal power, that is the driving force for change (see Chapter 5).

Energy itself may be a hindrance. Too much activity, when we fall out of rhythm with the world in which we live, can also bring about illness. While the energy debate relies upon vitalizing the sick, other healing traditions have based their explanations on energies that need to flow and be regulated (Lerner 1994).

Energy medicine

If we look at traditional Indian forms of medicine, Aryuveda and Unani (Greco-Arabian), we have a vitalist epistemology based upon the physician as activator of the seven natural principles which administer the body (elements, temperaments, humours, members, vital breaths, faculties and functions) (Verma and Keswani 1974). In this sense, after Hippocrates, 'Nature heals; the physician is nature's assistant.' Breath is an important factor in activating the patient. Vitality itself derives from *viva*, 'Let him live.' Such a living force is carried by the breath. Breath and spirit share the same root, in Latin *spirare*, which later becomes *spiritus*, literally life breathed in as a holy spirit. Life has the quality of inspiration and is heard in biblical texts as 'I am the Breath of Life.' Similarly the Greek *anemos* and the Latin *anima* are translated as wind and breath. Thus we have the ideas of vitality and animation being achieved through the inspiration of the breath, or *pneuma* in Unani medicine, which is the conveyor of the spirit (see Table 2.4) and activates, through its various parts, particular systems. Today Aryuvedic medicine, Chinese Qi-Gong and Yoga utilise the regulation of breathing as an important factor in healing through this process of activation. An explanation differing from physical science concepts that use the notion of work as energy, which is measurable.

Table 2.4 Breath and its activities		
Vital pneuma	Formed in the heart and conveyed through the arteries	All vital activities
Animal pneuma	Located in the brain and transported by the nerves	Intellect, sensation, dynamic and movement
Natural pneuma	Located in the liver and transported by the veins	Sensual desire, nutrition and blood formation

Benor, an American psychiatrist now resident in England who has made a detailed study of healing initiatives (Benor 1991), offers a definition of healing which succinctly combines most of the modern concepts found in spiritual healing. Healing is 'the intentional influence of one or more persons upon a living system without using known physical means of intervention' (p.9). In medicine, the original meaning of intentionality refers to the self-healing properties of wounds. These self-healing properties are multidimensional and include immune and hormonal responses and psychological factors within a social context. The etymological roots of intention are in the Latin *tendere* which means a stretching of the mind to become attentive, with expectation. This extended attention of the mind is a dynamic process of shifting awareness to the other as an offer of contact. Influence, from the Latin *influere*, is a flowing in. (Influenza, from the same root, is a malady caused by the flowing in, literally *in-fluence*, of heavenly bodies). Healing, from this perspective, is the offer of a dynamic process; the stretching of the mind of the healer which flows into the other person.

As part of everyday language in talking about illness we may describe one of the indicators that we are ill as listlessness or lack of energy. Indeed, doctors would not be surprised by the use of such language. A resumption to previous energy levels would itself be seen as recovery. Reported energy levels are a feature of assessing health profiles and some practitioners may go so far as to ask about the libido as an indicator of the general state of health. Energy talk has a value already when talking about health. However, it has become controversial when we begin to explain how healing works.

Healing touch

Several ancient healing techniques based on the conscious process of directing energies through a focus on the hands have been brought together in the use of therapeutic touch (Fischer and Johnson 1999).

Grad (Grad, Cadoret and Paul 1961) worked with a recognized 'healer', Oskar Estebany, the retired Hungarian army officer. Estebany was to be the inspiration for a variety of successful and elegant healing experiments with plants and mice, some of which were replicated (Solfin 1984). These experiments were carefully controlled and hastened growth or healing. Smith (1972), a Franciscan nun and biochemist worked with Estebany to test the hypothesis that any healing force channelled through or made active by the hands of a 'paranormal' healer must affect enzyme activity.

At first she compared the effects of laying on of hands by Estebany on the activity of the enzyme trypsin. Solutions of trypsin[1] were divided into four samples: one sample was an unaltered control state; one sample was treated by Estebany in the same way in which he treated patients by laying on hands;[2] another was exposed to ultraviolet light[3] for sufficient time to reduce the activity to 68–80 per cent (Grad had suggested that an 'unhealthy' enzyme be treated) and then treated by Estebany; one sample was exposed to a high magnetic field[4] for hourly increments for up to three hours.

The qualitative effect of a high magnetic field and a paranormal healer on the enzyme trypsin were similar and quantitatively the same, in that enzyme activity

---

1   500 ug per ml in 0.001 N HCI, pH3.

2   Putting his hands around a stoppered flask containing the enzyme solution for a maximum of 75 minutes from which 3 ml portions were pipetted out after 15,30,45 and 60 minutes.

3   2537 Ångstrom.

4   8–13,000 gauss.

increased up to one hour of exposure. Smith (1972) while warning against drawing too close a parallel between magnetic field effects and similar treatment effects from a healer, suggests that both forces bring about a change in organization of hydrogen bonding in the molecules bringing about a higher enzymic activity. It is this organizing force that is assumed to be the healing principle.

This work was repeated with three people who claimed to have no healing powers and three who did. They had no positive effect on the enzymes. Neither did Estebany when an attempt was made to replicate the experiment. His failure was attributed to his state of mind at the time not being conducive to healing. However, later three recognized healers were able to alter the enzyme according to spectro-photometric analysis in the way that Estebany had done. The quantitative effect varied daily according to the physical or emotional state of the healer. Further experiments with other enzymes[5] resulted in a decrease in activity or an inability to influence activity. Smith argues that for the amylose this was a good sign in that a change in the amylose-amylase balance would not be conducive to healing. In all Smith (1972) believes that the effect of laying on of hands on enzymes contributes to the healing process.

Therapeutic touch developed from observations that Dora van Gelder Kunz made of the healer Estebany and her belief that nurses could learn its approach for healing humans. Dolores Krieger, then Professor of Nursing at New York University, was charged with recording what happened and developed with Kunz the hand-healing approach (Krieger 1979). As a nurse researcher, Krieger took up the challenge to demonstrate healing by laying on of hands in living human beings rather than in the test tube. She made a series of before and after studies on human subjects. Like Smith before her, she was influenced by the work of Grad and Estebany. As the dependent variable she took haemoglobin values. Haemoglobin values did appear to respond to both Estebany in the initial experiments and to a small group of nurses whom Krieger trained in the art of laying on of hands (she called it 'therapeutic touch'). Furthermore, there is anecdotal evidence that the well-being of the patients improved.

Krieger's energetic approach follows the intentionality rationale offered by Benor earlier. Intentionality, as intelligent direction of energy, is seen as creating a pattern for healing. The person is seen as a collection of energy fields out of which patterns emerge. We see the same descriptions in ancient systems of spiritual healing where energy is described as vibrations. Where this energy description claims to be spiritual is that the form of energy itself is an exceedingly fine and subtle vibration. The energy fields of life would be open to such vibrational

5   Nicotinomide-adenine-dinucleotide and amylase-amylose.

influences, matter being a relatively coarse form of a slower vibration (Khan 1974). Some energy fields organize and influence other energy fields like magnetic forces influence iron filings and gravity exerts its influence on bodies. Healing touch, without actually touching the body, is supposed, by the conscious direction of the healer, to influence energy fields of the patient such that they achieve their own regulation. The role of the healer in this form of healing then is not to implement a cure but to activate 'through the healer's own love and compassion the healing potential within the patient' (Wirth 1993). As Smith had remarked, it is the ability of healers to organize and influence energy that is important.

The experimental evidence regarding therapeutic touch does not provide conclusive proof of energy exchange despite some extremely sophisticated and elegant research (Wirth 1995; Wirth *et al.* 1996a; Wirth and Cram 1997; Wirth, Richardson and Edelman 1996b). It is important to mention here that these experiments demonstrate the difficult in researching spiritual healing phenomena and, as we shall see in Chapters 6 and 7, this lies in the incompatibilities of the epistemologies that we use to describe healing and the methodological implications for conducting outcomes research based on those epistemologies.

Mind or matter: The epistemology of healing

Gregory Bateson (1978, 1991) argues that it is possible for us to be wrong about how we form our opinions and organize our descriptions in that the epistemology for healing – of forms and patterns – is different to that of hard science – of energy and matter. Mental processes are triggered by differences and that difference is not energy but information. Biological systems are organized by information, that is, significant differences rather than by forces or impacts. 'The letter that you do not write, the apology that you do not offer, the food that you do not put out for the cat' (Bateson 1978) contain no energy, but they do contain information. It is the world of thought which is of importance, because, as we are discovering, what people think and believe have implications for what they do. Mind affects matter. For example, I have no doubt infuriated the spiritual energy lobby by what I have written and the response may include elevated blood pressure or even vocal expressions. No 'energy' has been exchanged between the writer and the reader. Energy exchange is not necessary between self-energizing systems. However, energy release may have been triggered by words, which is a different dimension of interaction. Bateson also writes:

> If there are still readers who want to equate information and difference with energy, I would remind them that *zero* differs from *one* and can therefore trigger response, The starving amoeba will become more active, hunting for food; the growing plant will bend away from the dark, and the income tax people will

become alerted by the declarations you did not send. Events *which are not* are different from those which might have been, and events which are not surely contribute no energy. (Bateson 1978, p.111)

What the energy debate misses is the symbolic nature of the healing act and mirrors the blindness of natural science materialism. It is meaning in context, a cultural symbolic understanding, which is vital. This is not to deny energy but simply to locate energy within a context of meaning, which itself promotes a higher understanding and, as we have seen earlier, such a concept would be considered transcendental. What is important to remember here is that the term energy is being used both literally and as metaphor (Klivington 1997) and it is here that confusion often begins. As my friend George in Chapter 1 understood, the giving of blood that the other may have life had both a literal impact and a metaphoric meaning. While the transfer of blood cells had ramifications for his physical energy, those understandings he gleaned from the symbolic act were of a different realm of phenomena. As we shall see in Chapter 6, the laying on of hands in ritual healing is a symbolic act within a healing context, the experience of which has ramifications for those involved.

Transcendence as heresy

The notion of transcendence has always been a thorn in the side of established religion. For the mystic there is a way of direct knowing, indifferent to the world, that is inward and based upon personal revelation. Such personal knowledge dispenses with the hierarchies of priests as mediators dispensing knowledge and absolution to supplicants in need. Transcendent understanding is individual, internal and experiential as opposed to the external, institutional and scriptural dogma of established religion (Roof 1998). A paradox within the postmodern debate is that although an identity is sought that constitutes a unity with others, and particularly with nature, there is also a heightened sense of individuality and personal freedom that rejects any sense of external authority and a dislike of mainstream dogma (Bloch 1998). Long (1997) encourages patients and practitioners to discover their own definition of spirit and suggests that this will be free of religion and free from bias. This is a postmodern emphasis on the glorified liberated self and promotes extreme individuality blind to the cultural nexus in which the individual finds herself (see Table 2.5).

Table 2.5 Spirituality as postmodern	
Spirituality is regarded to be of human origin, not based on worship or creed, but paradoxically from something inherently within the self of a person, which symbolizes his or her spirituality in humanness. (p.500)	(Long 1997)
Spirituality means freely interacting with the world on the basis of a system of ultimate values and meanings, whatever the source of those meanings … it involves interacting with the world not merely thinking about the world; that is spirituality is concrete rather than abstract … the source of the ultimate values and meanings is not important. (p.31) Spirituality…is rule-governed behavior with the stipulation that the 'rule' is a belief that is evaluated as 'right' on the basis of a set of beliefs. (p.47)	(Reese 1997)
There is another dimension called the non-observable, which is the source of religion's purpose and meaning. It is the failure to recognize the difference between the observable and the non-observable, confusing the one with the other or by denying one in behalf of the other, that confounds our understanding of religion. (p.366)	(Idinopulos 1998)
Spirituality = any human practice which maintains contact between the everyday world and a more general meta-empirical framework of meaning by the way of individual manipulation of symbolic systems. (p.147)	(Hanegraaff 1999)

While transcendental knowledge may serve as the experiential basis for religious institutions, it has also functioned to challenge such institutions, thus heresy. In modern times, the sense of a personal identity has come to the fore and this has led to an individualized sense of reality, although that reality may be based on a cosmic totality. Individuals are searching for a sense of wholeness within a meta-physical context. In my previous work on suicidal behaviour, I referred to a similar process where individuals define themselves personally and within family contexts but also within broader cultural contexts. This broader cultural context of construing offers a variety of possible identities that challenges the previous religious and ethnic identities that were offered. We have a movement away from dogmas and creeds to a search for a personal identity that will be temporary and experienced as a means of personal expression. As we saw earlier, if there is a performance aesthetic to how people live their lives, then beliefs too are based upon action. Spirituality from this perspective is a way of becoming, engaging a challenging world through a developing self.

Language as sustaining

The difficulty of this individualistic approach is that we have no metaphysical sense of belonging. Once religious institutions are rejected, and they themselves become out of touch with everyday life, then we lose the language associated with them and their practices. For example, forgiveness is a central feature of many religions, but in its association with sin it may be seen as inappropriate to modern health care. However, some authors are realizing that forgiveness is what some people may need before healing can take place (Aponte 1998; Canale, White and Kelly 1996; Consoli 1996; Ferch 1998; Hargrave and Sells 1997; Pollard *et al.* 1998; Walrond-Skinner 1998). Central to this argument is that the language we use to talk about what concerns us and how we understand the world is vital. Language sustains us and the ability to use that language freely is an important part of our personal expression. The denial of such language is inhibiting. When patients are not allowed to talk of their spiritual concerns to their practitioners, then not only is important clinical information being missed but the patient is also being denied an aspect of his very being. As I wrote in Chapter 1, the importance of language is that it can be used within a community of users such that retains vitality and meaning. If we lose words like forgiveness, transcendence and grace from the vocabulary of healing, then we are in danger of impoverishing the very healing culture that we need.

With an emphasis on the personal, a pessimism regarding scientific progress and a scepticism to organized religion, where the old certainties are denied and rationality is seen as one of a variety of perceptions on an ever-shifting truth, then we have the stage set for understandings that are termed as postmodern.

A postmodern perspective

In the Enlightenment perspective which drives the modernist argument, knowledge is power and man possesses nature (Gillespie 1998). Such a perspective is no longer valid. Scientific progress is real, but also raises problems of mass destruction and pollution. Religions, while providing bastions of culture and succour to the poor, are also the wellsprings of major massacres.

The postmodern argument is principally a constructivist argument: that we, as human beings, construct the world in which we have our being and not some outside or higher power; a spirituality without a god or the divine but perhaps with a relationship to the forces and powers of nature. While seemingly postmodern, this is an extension of the modern argument that claims to have power over nature through reason. Where the postmodern debate diverges from the modern is that there a dialogue is entered into with nature (Wiesing 1994), but there is no one reasonable means of interpreting nature. Science and religion as grand interpretative narratives are gone. There is no attainable Truth but temporary, emergent and immanent truths that are experienced. There are no global utopias. God is dead, heaven has gone and we are spared the vagaries of hell. There are histories but no universal History. Illusions of unity are removed. Truth, reason, god, the divine, nature, all lose their capital letters.

How we understand the world depends upon the way in which we construct those understandings. They are no longer given to us from external authorities but are based on experiencing the world. The world is acted upon, not thought about but done. Thus, health is performed and is a process that is achieved. Like truth, health is immanent and emerges through action.

Belief in action

In the previous book about suicide I took the position that behaviour is rule governed. How we attribute meaning to events and how those events are acted upon follow constitutive and regulative rules that are interlocking levels of personal, relational and cultural construing. Reese (1997) also takes a rule-governed perspective on spirituality, stripping it to a minimal concept of a consistency of actions based on 'right' belief (see Table 2.5). Spirituality, as the opposite of materiality, or defined as the quest for ultimate meaning or the emotional experience of transcendence, is seen as too narrow. Spirituality involves acting in the world 'based on a system of ultimate values and meanings, whatever the source of those values and meanings. These may be religious doctrine, but it can equally well be success, power or sexual energy' (Reese 1997, p.31). Beliefs are deemed to be 'right' if they are based on freely adopted principles, not whether they conform to social norms but whether they form a consistent set of beliefs. Thus being a Christian freely would be different to being a Christian for its social benefits or to achieve political success. Beliefs must have a purpose rather than serve a purpose. The role of emotion is to provide the energy necessary for acting on those beliefs. What Reese fails to tell us is how those ultimate values and meanings are obtained, for if they are simply given then the argument is not postmodernism but modernism without the divine and without purpose.

What Reese's argument emphasizes is action: action based on belief; not only the willingness to do something but the importance of doing the thing itself. When our beliefs fail and the actions in which we engage are not consequent upon those beliefs, then we become alienated. There is an estrangement between ourselves and the world of others and we may even feel lost within ourselves. If what we do in everyday life has little personal meaning for us and we go through the motions of living without commitment, then we have a state of spiritual loss. This is what we saw in Chapter 1 with the woman who was grieving for her lost husband and felt that she had become alienated from her god. She was estranged not only from that other person with whom her life had made sense but also from any meaning and further purpose in her life.

While Eva's situation may have appeared as depression based upon grief, it reflects a situation found in many people who become suicidal. Their lives fail to make any further sense. They live beyond their psychological and personal resources. Everything they have is used up. This is the process of desertification. One way of changing is to transcend the current situation, not by thinking, but by doing. People who had been suicidal said that what made a difference was not formalized counselling but doing things differently: planting a garden in spring; buying new curtains; being given a cat to look after (Aldridge 1998). Small practical steps bring about realizations of another truth and this has been the emphasis of many religions on techniques for realizing the truth, through ritual, prayer and meditation. Idinopulus (1998) refers to religion as 'energy, faith, a vision of transcendence, and the will to live in relation to it' (p.376).

No unity

A postmodern reality is not unified. There are multiple clamouring voices, each of which is justified. Our challenge is to make sense of such diversity and a sense that will be temporary and fragile. This process of interpretation is aesthetic, in that it is based on styles of constituting the world, and pragmatic, in that the world has to be done. We regulate our actions based on what we believe. Such diversity is seen in the delivery of health care and how we talk about health and illness, as we shall see in Chapter 4. We already have a plurality of approaches in health-care delivery with surgery, internal medicine, psychosomatics, psychology, psychiatry, acupuncture, dietary approaches, homeopathy and chiropractic. The beliefs on which these practices are based are not accidental. They belong to cultural construings that are consistent among a community of believers and practitioners. Doctors, scientists, healers, as well as patients, have their beliefs and practices that are regular and consistent. In modern health care there is a demand for health-care outcomes as if there was a unity in those beliefs and practices as to what constitutes health or healing. Such outcomes will be impossible. What we can compare is consequences of healing based upon consistency of actions predicated on belief systems. Thus pharmaceutical treatments will have differing outcomes compared with spiritual interventions simply because the consequence of actions is based upon differing sets of beliefs. One set of outcomes does not negate the others, but to expect each to conform to a common set of outcomes is illusory and maintains that both have a unified belief system which determines actions. We see this reflected in the fruitless search to validate spiritual healing in terms of material outcomes. One approach to reality, spiritual healing, seeks to validate its consequences upon the beliefs of a different order of a material reality, and fails.

A challenge to science

The profanity of science is that it attempts to predict and control by human agency, whereas the spiritual brings that which is new and sacred by 'divine agency' or 'nature'. That this agency is described as emerging from within the person or occurring externally to that person depends upon his religion and its culture of discerning knowledge. The best empirical scientific methods for understanding are simply not the best methods for understanding the impact of spirituality. Empiricism is that which is understood through the senses and thereby material. Frithjof Schuon (1989) writes: 'We must not also abase things which transcend us, for then our virtue loses all its value and meaning; to reduce spirituality to a "humble utilitarianism" – that is, to a kind of materialism – is to cast aspersions on God' (p.120).

What we learn more and more is that in our search for regularities, then we discover irregularity. That this irregularity, like the weather, also has a pattern is a transcendent understanding. A yardstick of science is Occam's razor, that there is elegance in simplicity. This metaphor has been superseded as science must also leave its classical roots and the Greek mythologies that inform its metaphors.

We now have the era of the fractal, the repeated pattern of complexity, not simplicity, at endless levels. In the face of complexity, we do not have to retreat into superstition or oversimplification. We can focus on the patient before us and how she makes sense of the world through the story she tells us. Sometimes we 'lose the plot'. Our narratives fail us, faith in our beliefs is lost. We are no longer sure about the directions we are taking. We ask questions about the ideals that we once had when we were young. This is the human condition and perhaps when we realize that illness is the questioner. In those moments when we begin to question, through doubt or pain, then the argument about which truth is not so important as how we come to acquaint ourselves with truth: not what we believe, but how we believe. This is what unites practitioner and patient in the search for healing.

Knowledge and its consequences

In this way we share our knowledge. We have shared understandings. This is not knowledge to win an argument, as we have in academia or within medical debates either complementary or orthodox, but knowledge that takes us further. We speak and listen to each other, not in combat but in a purposive dialogue of understanding. How we hold differing narratives together is the challenge to patients and practitioners. The way in which we treat each other with compassion and understanding affects our professional and personal lives. Knowledge has its consequences. In this way, institutions will have to meet the needs of patients and staff, not the person having to fit the institution. These are the consequences of a pragmatics of action based on belief not dogma.

Even within modern medicine we have difficulty in defining health. Bateson (1991) reminds us of the relationship between the sacred and health. He writes that it is difficult to talk about living systems that are doing well; it is easier to describe those systems when they are disturbed. Thus parts are separated from the whole and the necessary connection between those parts is lost. This restoring of connection, the making of the completed whole, is the task for which we are prepared as practitioners and healers, yet eludes our descriptions as scientists and researchers. With George in Chapter 1, we began to see how connections were restored at other levels, although the connections within his material body were lost. In some ways we act as if pain, suffering, illness and death were not to be expected in life. While we may strive for the eradication of major diseases, the presence of suffering will be a part of the human narrative; so too then, the relief of that suffering. How that relief is achieved will not be dependent solely upon a medical narrative but, as the major religions have offered throughout the ages, also upon spiritual understanding.

Coda

In the next chapter I shall go on to offer a series of definitions of religion. These definitions overlap with those of spirituality. If spirituality is about the individual, ineffable and implicit, religion is about the social, spoken and explicit. Such definitions are an attempt to explicate the practices whereby spirituality is achieved.

Spirituality lends meaning and purpose to our lives and these purposes help us transcend what we are. We are processes of individual development in relational contexts, that are embedded within a cultural matrix. We are also developing understandings of truth. Indeed, each one of us is an aspect of truth. These understandings are predicated on changes in consciousness achieved through transcending one state of consciousness to another. This dynamic process of transcendence is animated by forces or subtle energies. For some authors these energies are organized as information or energies that organize energies. It is at this level of organization that we have a connection to the spiritual traditions which talk of levels of vibrations and an intelligence within the universe as higher knowledge. If science studies the gradual process of entropy, the dissolution of order in the universe, then spirituality studies the opposing process of negentropy, the movement out of chaos into order. If technology is the means by which science is made real, then religion is the *techne* of spirituality.

In terms of healing, spirituality encourages a change in consciousness such that the current situation can be transcended. How this is translated into concrete heath-care terms is problematic. For the worried, there may be release from temporal concerns. For the anxious, there may be comfort. For the dying, they will see purpose. For those in pain, there may be relief. For the chronically sick, there may be hope. But when we look for concrete manifestations then they are elusive and not predictable at a level of straightforward correspondence. We are not going to see an immediate relief of suffering in all instances. There are enough stories of spiritual masters dying from everyday diseases after years of sickness. Death may be a negative end-point for modern medicine, but from a spiritual perspective it will simply be release from a physical bond. At a mundane level, symptoms may persist, disabilities may remain, but how they are experienced and handled in everyday life may change. When spiritual healing tries to remove such symptoms or bring about concrete changes, the results are not always predictable. The lack of predictability of spiritual healing lies in the material expectations of the observers and misses the point of what spirituality leads us to understand. It is precisely this 'missing the point' that in spiritual teachings is regarded as the concept of 'sin'. 'Sin' is simply missing the point, not understanding.

A sense of purpose in life may emerge despite a continuing illness. Hope can vibrate in lives that may be severely limited. It is possible to transcend loss and live a life of renewed vigour and peaceful contemplation. Identifying with a conscious and unified universe may put our everyday concerns into another perspective. The will to live may be capricious for some and renewed spontaneously for others, but few of us would want to invalidate its benefits for health. How that will to live manifests itself will be individually achieved according to the purpose of that person's life and the developmental needs necessary for achieving understanding of that purpose. Thus, we would anticipate a change in consciousness, a new understanding of a personal truth and how that relates to other truths. If each one of us is a living truth in itself, then other truths are achieved through relationship. If the world as we meet it is a series of lived truths, then it is through this encounter with a living universe that we expand knowledge. Science will be one way of structuring this encounter through sets of rituals, official texts, belief systems, creeds and practices. Religion will offer us another. However, in the end, an understanding of spirituality is that it re-establishes a contact between the human and the divine. This is the unity of consciousness, a becoming whole and the basis of the healing endeavour.

3

Religion
The everyday forms of spiritual life

Essentially religion has two roles, which in all surviving systems has become confused through the absence of specialist knowledge in the publicists and most visible and active theoreticians. The first is to organise man in a safe, just and peaceful manner to help maintain communities. The second is the inner aspect, which leads people from the outward stabilisation to the performance which awakens them and makes them permanent. (Idries Shah 1971)

The poetry and the teaching to which you have referred is an outward manifest-ation. You feed on outward manifestation. Do not, please, give that the name of spirituality. (Quoted in the story of 'The Cook's Assistant', Idries Shah 1969)

From the literature related to spiritual healing in medical and nursing contexts that we saw in the previous chapter, there appears to be an emerging consensus that the term religious is used as an operationalization or outward manifestation of 'spirituality' (see Table 3.1). There are spiritual practices in which people engage that often take place in groups and are guided by culture. As a cultural system, religion is a meaning seeking activity that offers the individual and others both purpose and an ability to perceive meaning. We have not only a set of offered meanings but also the resources and practices by which meanings can be realized. However, as Idries Shah reminds us in the above quote, we must be wary of confusing 'spirituality' with what is manifested outwardly.

Many writers say that religious experiences are organized to mediate the flux of human experience. Religion achieves this mediation through practices like prayer and worship. It often offers an exemplary grounded myth about the illustrative life of a prophet, which in literate societies will be written as a text. There will be a code of ethical practice and a series of ritual processes. When such practices are organized as a stable system over time then we see the emergence of 'churches' in a community.

Table 3.1 Religion as belief operationalized as practices

The term religiousness has been used in operationalizing spirituality. (p.336)	(Reed 1987)
By religious we mean practices carried out by those who profess a faith. (p.303)	(Doyle 1992)
The term religious will be used to denote the part of the process when spiritual impulses are formally organized into a social/political structure designed to facilitate and interpret the spiritual search. (p.34)	(Decker 1993)
Religion has a beneficial effect on human social life and individual well-being because it regulates behaviour and integrates individuals in caring social circles. (p.684)	(Idler 1995)
Religion is considered by some to be of divine origin with a set of revealed truths and a form of worship. (p.500)	(Long 1997)
Religion is or has been a response to socially induced vulnerability, it is and always has been a response to the physical vulnerability of the body that has been the human condition. (p.648)	(Walter and Davie 1998)
Religion will not be defined in strict terms, but will be used to denote experiences, cognitions and actions seen (by the individual or the community) as significant in relation to the sacred. (p.260)	(Ganzevoort 1998)
Religiosity is associated with religious organizations and religious personnel... Religion involves subscribing to a set of beliefs or doctrines that are institutionalized... People...can be religious without being spiritual by perfunctorily performing the necessary rituals. However, in many cases, spiritual experiences do accompany religious practices. (p.65)	(Lukoff *et al.* 1999)
Religion is the outward practice of a spiritual system of beliefs, values, codes of conduct and rituals. (p.1259)	(King and Dein 1998)
Religion encompasses that which is designated by the social group as nonroutine and uncontrollable and that which inspires fear, awe, and reverence, that is, the sacred. Through ritual, one gains carefully prescribed access to the sacred, which is carefully protected from the mundane, routine, instrumentally oriented beliefs and actions of the profane realm. Because sacredness is socially confirmed, stemming from the attitude of believers... political ideologies, value systems and even leisure activities such as sports and art (are viewed) as sacred activities. (p.407)	(Park 1998)

These religious practices also regulate social interaction and sometimes have specific requirements for dress and prohibitions regarding diet. We will see such requirements concerning lifestyle and their link to health-care practices in the next chapter. The traditional role of religion has been a unified way of organizing life, where deities are invoked to regulate the vagaries of daily living, rules are instilled for appropriate social conduct and dietary prohibitions are imparted according to the needs of tribal hygiene. What unifies this world of events is an overarching culture of symbolism such that meaning can be discerned in day-to-day activity. Thus religious dietary practices may be about feeding, as nutrition, but are also symbolic. Specific foods are used symbolically in rituals of marriage, death, festivals and special gatherings (Grivetti *et al.* 1987). Yet there are also possible health-care benefits from food prohibitions. The avoidance of pork lessens trichinosis. Abstention from stimulants among Mormons and meat among Seventh Day Adventists leads to stronger and healthier life (Levin and Schiller 1987). Anthroposophy offers a detailed agricultural practice based on organic crop production that, if followed, would have prevented the current problems concerning the contamination of meat products. Religions have traditionally offered a cultural system for daily living, offering resources for discovering meaning and purpose, stabilizing communities and maintaining identity. Even with a shift towards subjectivity in postmodern societies, that individualism is still contextualized within social networks or small-scale communities. Indeed, the danger of postmodernism is that it may promote a retreat into tribalism or an alienated individualism (Aldridge 1996).

Durkheim saw these cultural interpretations as secondary. There is an implicit importance to the social nature of religion for human thought that is fundamental. Socially enacted events provide the shared ideas that form the basis of the human intellect. Implicit in the practice of religion is a moral force that is discernible to the individual as feeling achieved through participation in social practice (Rawls 1996a, 1996b). Social practices, like religion, give rise to feelings of unity that come to mind as whole and not from internal analysis. This is different to the sensation of natural events through the senses of smell, sight, touch, taste and hearing. Reason receives its form from the real world of the social. While we are biological individuals, we achieve our human understanding through social practices and these categories of understanding, as a framework, shape our perceptions. Thus the spiritual feeling of unity that we saw in the previous chapter would be engendered as a 'feeling' through the social, even though it may be interpreted as personal revelation. Such feelings are dependent upon enacted social practice. It is precisely such emotionalism that Shah says is not spirituality (Shah 1977). It may engage people in religious satisfactions but is not to be confused with the development of consciousness.

From this Durkheimian perspective, it is not a universe of symbols that shape thought and action. There are categories of understanding, space, time, class, force, causality and totality that arise out of social action and are the prerequisite for the cultural. Cultural symbols are specific interpretations of basic categorical understandings. As Rawls (1996a) writes: 'The collective representations come, at least indirectly, from the categories that in turn come from 'feelings' which are apprehensions by participants of moral forces generated during social practice.' While the individual will observe phenomena and have a sense of regularity from those observations, they remain individual, subjective and incommunicable. By participating in the social group, we are offered a framework in which those experiences can arrange themselves, which allows us to think about them and to say them and communicate with each other. Shared practice is the source of shared knowledge that is perceived as feeling. This knowledge is truth and reason and must be transmitted. People are not free to construct ideas in whatever way they wish. There has to be a social intelligibility. Action defines meaning and social action, as practice, fulfils social needs. This action provides a real moral force occurring within society. We saw this in the previous chapter, where some healers will refer to force and energy in their debate about how spiritual healing works. This may be a direct example of a Durkheimian direct feeling of moral force in the individual through the social action of a healing ritual. Any material efforts to measure such events would be totally misplaced, as are explanations that seek an empirical validation at the physiological level. The phenomenon is social. As we shall see later in this chapter, it is religious actions by faith communities that offer new understandings through social action. However, the action itself is still social, religious but not spiritual.

Finding a sense of meaning

When faced with chaos and death we become anxious. If we fail to understand our experiences then our personal lives lose their meaning. We are threatened with lives that have no purpose, no sense of direction, and we lose our connection to those with whom our lives make sense. The primary need is to find some sense of coherent meaning that offers an internal consistency of purpose and identity and an external coherence that unites us with those others with whom we share our daily lives. By maintaining some coherence in current meaning, then we link the present to the past and can contemplate the future. This has been the role of religion: to provide a stable set of meanings such that an ultimate ordering of the universe can be cultivated and whereby a link to the sacred, the uncontrollable, can be made (Ganzevoort 1998; Park 1998).

Meanings are not only given, but are also linked to practices like meditation and prayer such that meanings can be revealed. Thus religious meanings have the potential to be revived according to a changing cultural context. A scientist discovers new meanings through the questioning process of research. A disciple discovers new meanings through the process of prayer and worship. A contemplative discovers new meanings through the process of meditation. An artist discovers new meanings through painting. Each, from her own perspective, has a technology of discovery. Each is seeking her own particular set of knowledge such that her life can be lived appropriately.

A revealed set of truths is effective when it is pertinent to the context in which the person lives. An emphasis on practices that encourage the discovery of meaning, while being a threat to priestly classes which attempt to control meaning for their own purposes of power, means that understandings can be made that are appropriate for each new generation. As Shah (1990) suggests, the point in considering religion and its manifestations is not to turn us into medieval sages but twentieth-century beings capable of making intelligible decisions. We can say the same of religious healing. Rather than turn us into besandalled disciples setting out with nothing more than a satchel, we need to develop an intelligence that can discern the heath-care needs of those within the communities we serve. This discernment will necessitate an awareness of current medicines as the basis of health-care delivery, which includes economic considerations and also religious understandings such that health-care delivery is coherent with the identities of persons in the relevant communities.

Constructing meaning

Health care, if it is to make any inroads into tackling the burgeoning problems of suffering in modern-day life, will need to consider the systems by which people construct meaning within their lives. Both religion and medicine have related interests: their regard for fundamental principles concerning the meaning and sanctity of human life (Perrett 1996); the interplay between body and mind (Campbell 1998); and the meaning of suffering and sickness (Vanderpool and Levin 1990). These commonalities come to the fore in current debates about the sanctity of life in abortion, the response to genetic defects in fetal anomalies (Calhoun, Reitman and Hoeldtke 1997), surrogate motherhood, alternative forms of fertilization, sterilization (Miller and Finnerty 1996) and genetic manipulation. We also discuss end of life issues related to unnecessary suffering (Long 1997; Roy 1996) and euthanasia (Bartholome 1996). On another level, we debate the availability of health-care delivery: who is to be treated in terms of social justice; what is to be treated, as in male impotence; and what is necessary to treat and reimburse, in terms of cosmetic surgery. There are also legal implications like treating children against the will of their parents or blood transfusions in the face of religious prohibitions (Frohock 1993).

While modern medicine attempts to argue its scientific basis and encourages us to believe that it should be solely evidence based, it is plain to the non-involved observer that decisions concerning the sanctity of life, the struggle with death and the value of the individual are also elements to be found within religion. That medicine itself is purely scientific and can be practised on the grounds of available research is as much a dogma as we would find in any organized religion, and as much a matter of faith. Given that faith is a mixture of belief and emotion, then the style in which some practitioners defend their medical enterprise disqualifies their stance as purely scientific. We have a culture informed by science and religion and understanding how the two complement each other is vital. As Gregory Bateson writes:

> Mere purposive rationality unaided by such phenomena as art, religion, dream and the like, is necessarily pathogenic and destructive of life; and that its virulence springs specifically from the circumstance that life depends upon interlocking circuits of contingency, while consciousness can only see such short arcs of such circuits as human purpose may direct. (Bateson 1978, p.118)

Our task is to learn how each arc of the circle of understanding unites with other arcs to complete the whole circle and thus enhance each other for the benefit of those partaking. Csordas (1983) criticizes both religion and medicine for failing to generate those integrative accounts of the same phenomena that occur in the process of healing.

Social integration

A modern sociological perspective on religion sees it as beneficial for human social life and well-being (see Table 3.2). It integrates the individual within a social caring milieu (Durkheim 1995), offers a set of meanings for understanding personal and cosmic events (Weber 1964) and provides a symbolic universe where events gain significance (Berger 1967). If personal meanings are constructed, religion offers a cultural set of construings as a framework within which personal understandings can be accommodated. New Age movements and newer religions are demanding rules based lifestyle approaches to attract members (Park 1998) and the symbolic nature of myths, rituals, clothing and food is being emphasized. In addition, it is an understanding of the sacred as being uncontrollable, but being discernible, intelligible and having coherence that is placing nature once more in a prominent position for those New Age groups. Where the modern endeavour was for science to tame nature through technology, that project has been abandoned. Living in harmony with nature is seen as the basis for new religious perspectives. Unfortunately this can bring a swing, either real or imagined, that is interpreted as opposition to science. What we face is the challenge of incorporating our scientific understandings within a sacred consciousness which promotes the necessary intelligibility that we need for the coming century. This is not against science, it simply relativizes a scientific perspective. Marx saw religious suffering as an expression by the oppressed as 'of real suffering and a protest against suffering. Religion is the sigh of the oppressed creature, the feeling of a heartless world and the soul of soulless circumstances. It is the opium of the people' (Marx 1964).

Table 3.2 Religion as meaning	
In fact, re-ligio, from its roots, implies that 'foundation wall' to which one is bound for one's survival, the basis of one's being. (p.444)	(Sims 1994)
Religious life is an expressive, world-building activity through which we get ourselves together and find a kind of posthumous, or retrospective, happiness. (p.xiv)	(Cupitt 1997)
A religion is a shared view into the heart of the world, a perspective into the truth, but a perspective that is always also a veil. It is, moreover, not *just* a view or a perspective; it is a perspective that faces up to the fundamental mystery of the world more or less well. (p.550)	(Gillespie 1998)
Religion is a comprehensive picturing and ordering of human existence in nature and the cosmos. (p.220)	(Joseph 1998)
Religion = any symbolic system which influences human action by providing possibilities for ritually maintaining contact between the everyday world and a more general meta-empirical framework. (p.147)	(Hanegraaff 1999)

Medicine and its symbols

Medicine too offers us understandings about what it means to fall ill and how we can recover, how living and dying can be regulated through specific practices, how new life can be encouraged, how those lives can be developed and how lives can be protected from the vagaries of man and nature. We find, as in religion, a symbolic universe of medicines, dress codes, areas designated for healing and for research, with established institutions, including designated texts, and their hierarchies of practitioners and teachers.

The Greek god Asklepios, son of Apollo, symbolized a unity of medicine and religion. He was also the patron of physicians and protected them. His symbol, the snake-entwined staff, is still evident among some medical institutions on their letterheads or on the title pages of their journals. As the myth goes, he learned the healing arts from the wise centaur Chiron. Some of his children, Hygieia, Iaso, Akeso, Panakeia and Telesphoros represent personifications of the healing powers (Compton 1998). His sacred animals were the serpent, as found in his symbol representation today, and the dog. They symbolized an unconscious force that stirred below the surface of the waking world representing eternity, continuity and health (Angeletti *et al.* 1992).

Asklepios was also a central god to a caste of initiated priests who preserved a mysterious tradition of healing and he was a deity that restored health, as a sign of grace, to those who visited his temple. There were health centres founded on this deity throughout the time of the Roman emperors, situated in places where there was fresh spring water, fresh air and a benign climate, rather like modern day health spas and cure resorts.

In these resorts, those who were sick would pray, offer sacrifices and religiously purify themselves by bathing. The patients were often those whose illnesses had not submitted to the available medical initiatives (Compton 1998). There were designated places where the patient would enter into a dreamlike state between sleeping and waking and the divinity would appear to them. This appearance could be in the form of a snake or dog. Angeletti *et al.* (1992) suggests that this healing was not only symbolic but also exploited biological properties. There were factors in saliva that encouraged wound healing, for example, epidermal growth factor. We have, therefore, a mixture of symbolic and biological factors. As we saw in the previous chapter, there is not only a metaphoric character to religious healing, in this sense, but also a biological reality. Both combine to provide a rich complexity that some practitioners are demanding of modern day health care; not a return to the snakes and dogs of ancient temples, but a consideration of the symbolic and the biological that is the complex of healing.

A repertoire of symptoms

When we consider the symptom as it is presented, that symptom needs to be interpreted. If we only have one set of interpretations and this restricts the repertoire of treatment, then we significantly impoverish the healing culture that we present to our patients. A coherent network of symbols attached to experiences of falling ill and recovery, to the expression of distress and its relief, allow new meanings to be constructed and for new repertoires of healing to take place. As reflected in the ancient Greek and Roman periods of Asklepian treatment, medical initiatives fail when they do not meet the challenges of living in their existential breadth. As we saw in the previous suicide book, the impoverishment of treatment choices and a desertification of resources that occurs when distress fails to be reduced leads to an escalation in that distress and ultimately to suicide (Aldridge 1998). When patients were offered new meanings and simple actions then their recovery ensued. Distress was transcended by simple actions like planting bulbs in the garden with the promise of spring and new growth. This is both an actual and symbolic reality; so too with spiritual and religious healing.

If we fail to offer our patients an enriched symbolic world, then small wonder that they turn to medical alternatives which are more satisfying. Few writers have considered that perhaps it is the symbolic world of Chinese medicine, based upon vitalist explanations of a flowing energy, that in itself is attractive and makes sense in terms of healing. This is quite rightly a rejection of modern scientific medicine if it fails to meet the symbolic needs of the patient.

A symptom when presented is not simply an objective reality. The very fact that it is a symptom means that interpretation is necessary and symptoms too are symbolic of the process of distress. Relief of that distress must also achieve a symbolic understanding, thus a turn to religious and spiritual healing. Religious healing offers a symbolic world of integration beyond a cure. This is not to deny scientific medicine, but rather to highlight the impoverishment of health-care delivery which fails to understand that scientific medicine alone is wanting when we talk about health-care needs. Similarly, the healing initiatives that seek their validity in quantitative outcome research also impoverish this symbolic under-standing by seeking explanations at the inappropriate level of understanding.

In a pluralistic approach, we will offer a variety of interpretations and congruent treatments with meaningful processes of recovery that can be experi-enced. Each of these will have their own basis in evidence of recovery and the nature of that evidence needs to be established and discussed to find a com-monality of understanding.

Religious meaning as welfare and refuge

It is the social integrative aspect of religion that offers health-care benefits for the poor and the elderly. Traditionally offering succour to the weak and infirm has been an injunction of religious movements and resulted in varying initiatives for providing welfare throughout the nineteenth century. These have resulted in hospitals and hospices. Religious communities offer human comfort and sympathy within a framework of activities like worship, pastoral care, health-care initiatives and welfare projects. Distress is reduced within a community and such communities also offer alternative means of coping with health-care problems for individuals (Bienenfeld et al. 1997; Idler 1995; Musick et al. 1998; Pargament and Park 1995; Worthington et al. 1996).

Welfare for the poor is itself symbolic of the relationship of the divine, that is the 'all powerful' meeting the needs of the weakest. It is perhaps important to remark here that this meeting of welfare needs is as important for the giver as it is for the receiver. This is not consumerism, but a form of mutuality that brings spiritual benefits for the giver as well as for the receiver. Both are benefited within a common symbolic system of understandings. In this way the idea of charity was developed. Originally charity was meant to indicate a stage along the spiritual path and was anonymous, not the modern day expression of individual largesse to gain personal benefit for the giver too.

Social networks and health

Although physical disabilities or poor health may continue for the individual, a sense of personal worth and acceptance within a group of others as offered by a religious community has ramifications for well-being. An enhanced social net-work and an increased satisfaction with life may result in an improved health status. Self-ratings of health may be relatively positive despite serious or chronic illness (Idler 1997; Idler and Kasl 1997). Idler (1995) interviewed randomly selected clients of an urban rehabilitation clinic. These 146 clients were suffering with arthritis. They had a heterogeneous background of religious beliefs and practices. The intention of the study was to discern the impact of religious life on health-care outcomes and the influence such a lifestyle had on a personal sense of self.

Respondents with poorer health were more likely to have sought help from religion. Those who thought of themselves as strongly religious were more likely to say that they had received help from religion (Idler 1995, p.692). The more disabled people were, the more likely they were also to seek such help. Poorer health then is associated with religiosity. Religiosity is seen as an innate characteristic having two forms (Levin and Schiller 1987). An institutionalized form emphasizes collective experience and objectively observable phenomena often associated with affiliation to an organization such as a church. Interiorized religiosity is subjective and individual characterized by idiosyncratic beliefs or 'faith'.

When Idler interviewed the clients in his study, a non-physical sense of self, expressed as a spiritual dimension, was associated with higher levels of religiosity, better self-ratings of health and a possible higher level of education. A qualitative perspective showed that the stories people told reflected self-identities being enhanced by religious criteria. Illness events, like a stroke, were seen as dramatic events by the survivors proposing a moment of spiritual awakening that itself promoted a growth in spiritual life despite a restriction in physical capacity. This non-physical understanding was expressed as a discovery of the purpose of life and a sense of gratitude for being alive. We saw how a sense of life's purpose that transcended a current situation was an indicator of spirituality in the previous chapter. Death may indeed have lost some of its sting for those that come nearer to it through a stroke. It also gives us grounds to contemplate when we consider the research aspects of spiritual healing. Despite a negative outcome in physical ability, and physical ability is foremost in general health care, we see a change that is experienced as positive in terms of an enhanced sense of non-physical self. Healing may not be that which is asked for. There may be peace but no physical change or reconciliation may occur between family members but the patient still dies.

Gratitude for living was also extended to the work of the medical staff involved, who were seen as carrying out their work under a divine provenance. Sometimes clinicians and patients expect that religion and medicine must be kept separate. Yet in the daily lives of these clients there was pragmatic unity of both. Doctors were seen to be guided by the same divine presence that enabled the client to see in his illness the future needs of his life. What is necessary to see is that the tasks allotted to doctor and priest, while separate in practice, are not so easily separated in the patient's experience. I am not arguing here for doctors to take on the task of priests, nor priests becoming doctors. Rather that both understand each other and that for the benefit of the patient and his recovery there is some perspective of a unified soul. While our tasks are separate we do belong, doctor, priest and patient, to one community of healing. Although we are many, we are one body (Aldridge 1987).

In the same study, clients also talked about suffering as it related to religious beliefs. Spiritual understandings may not bring a material change or correspond directly to improvements in health care. People spoke of suffering that brought a sense of meaning, but no tangible physical healing or emotional comfort. Suffering was seen as a learning experience. Prayers were not seen as a practice that would necessarily have a direct material result. Indeed, the reflective process of praying and not gaining an answer was seen as having a benefit in that the person praying was to search deeper for a sense of meaning. Prayer in this sense is a religious practice that enables a spiritual understanding.

King and his colleagues reached a similar conclusion (King, Speck and Thomas 1994). Patients with a religious and spiritual life view who expressed strong beliefs 'were less likely to do well clinically' (p.635). However, it may have been that while disabilities were increased there was a corresponding growth in a non-physical sense of self. In a previous study, King, Speck and Thomas (1994) found a poorer outcome for those with strong religious beliefs or a spiritual view on life. The team at the Royal Free Hospital in London looked initially at 300 participants and assessed them using the general health questionnaire. There was a variety of illnesses, 50 per cent being related to heart and circulatory problems. While strength of religious belief is seen as predictive for health outcomes, it is important to understand that patients with a strongly expressed belief in a religious or spiritual life had poorer clinical outcomes.

Once we believe that prayer is efficacious in the process of healing, we must be wary of reducing those prayers to a material level. In a supportive religious context suffering can bring about a change in consciousness. How long that will take and how such change will be manifested is not amenable to prediction. We see this in the numerous healing studies that offer glimpses of significance following prayer. The problem is that such studies have narrow ends and determined time frames; the subtle is expected to conform to the gross. It is the nature of clinical research that we fix time points for recovery and deliberate about what recovery will look like as dependent variables. What we can do is to change our expectations about the nature of healing and what we take as evidence in terms that healing has occurred. Physical effects will occur, but we must also be aware of internal changes to the person that are subtle causes. Peace may be discovered although pain may not be significantly reduced. There may be reconciliation within a family with an elderly relative, but the dementia progresses degeneratively. Perhaps we can learn from the patients who saw through the process of suffering that there was a unity to all the healing endeavours. Medical interventions were also for them the manifestation of a divine presence or superior power (see Table 3.3).

Table 3.3 Religion as relationship between humans and a supernatural power or force	
Religion refers to faith, beliefs, and practices that nurture a relationship with a superior being, force or power. (p.43)	(Emblen 1992)
One definition…regards religion as a source of shared norms and values. This approach stresses the motive of belonging and the role of integrating the community system. Another definition…regards religion as the relationship between human beings and a postulated supranatural sphere of power. This approach stresses the motive of empowerment and the role of religion in legitimating societal authority. Religion may be part of the political system or a resource of power for the social agent. (p.250)	(Riis 1998)

Spirituality and religion

Modern authors (King and Dein 1998; Lerner 1994; Lukoff *et al.* 1999) have insisted that spirituality and religion can be separated, albeit with difficulty. Where spirituality is seen as subjective, religion is seen as being social and means subscribing to a set of doctrines that are institutionalized. Thus some people may be spiritual in that they have a sense of being related to the sacred but do not take part in any organized religion. Conversely, others may perform the expected rituals of religious observance but have no personal experience of the divine.

VandeCreek and colleagues (1999), in considering alternative therapies used by breast cancer patients, came to a similar conclusion. It is difficult to separate out the 'spiritual' variables from those associated with religious practices. Prayer, a traditional religious practice, is seen as being of major interest for 84.5 per cent of the breast cancer outpatients, alongside which 75.8 per cent show an interest in exercise, 48.3 per cent in spiritual healing and 47.4 per cent in relaxation, with a similar percentage interested in megavitamins. What becomes clear is that while we as academics in health care have a need for precision in delineating variables and a consistency of world view, our patients in their daily lives have less of a need for such epistemological abstemiousness and more of a pragmatic need for what can be done. Perhaps a decisive point is that this need for practice entails what the individual can do for her own recovery, not simply what the practitioners alone can do. Rather than swing between practitioner care and patient self-help as opposing entities, we may view health care like the patients in the rehabilitation study mentioned previously, as a joint endeavour.

Ganzevoort (1998) writes that religious behaviour is important for coping with crises. Maintaining an identity is an important factor for coping with the demands that life makes of us. Coping is a search for significance in times of stress and this has an obvious connection with the need for a personal sense of worth and meaning. Church attendance, for example, not only has a social function in providing support but also offers a lifestyle perspective. Prayer can promote solidarity with others and dedication to a common identified purpose. The ritualized structure of church services and planned liturgy offer some form of order in otherwise fragmented lives. Religion also offers sets of shared meanings that attempt to make sense of the vagaries of the world, a framework of disciplined feelings in which those meanings can find expression, and forms of expression in worship and prayer for feelings and belief within a regulated social setting. Religious practice in terms of healing may be easier to understand when we see that it makes spiritual understandings available as cognitions (beliefs), feelings (faith) and actions (prayer) that promote a coherent personal identity that can be maintained with a community of significant others.

Fabrega (1997) discusses the evolution of sickness and healing. He defines sickness as the socially constructed expression of a subjective state of illness and healing as the socially constructed efforts, procedures and medicines aimed at neutralizing illness. If disease is physiological, then sickness and healing are social and cultural (p.26). Showing and responding to disease and injury is a biological trait. Yet, healing in family-level societies is a public affair. Serious problems are mediated by ritual healing in groups that are open to public participation. Healing in this sense is part of the moral economy of a group and has value for social exchange, demonstrating a component of altruism that entails reciprocity at a time in the future. Thus religious healing in church groups is maintaining public participation for the moral economy of a community that is threatened by the individualism of advanced capitalism.

A sense of identity

A central feature of religion is the maintenance of a coherent sense of self and adherence to religious beliefs is a part of that coherent identity. However, a religious identity is related also to a transcendent object or divine being (see Table 3.3). What religious activities offer for those in crisis is a set of practices that support the questioner in her questioning at such times. Crisis is being used here in its broad sense of a time of judgement when discernment is required. This presupposes not only a cognitive and emotional response, but also a consequent act based on thoughts and feelings.

Some religious organizations may offer a set of ready-made answers at times of crisis. These answers are intended as a comforting preliminary stage according to the requirement of the questioner in her immediate need. They may also, however, be evidence of a religious context that has lost its spiritual vitality and has become corrupted as a set of superstitions. As those who work with the dying and their families are aware, how satisfying our answers are to the questioner lies in the stage of the questioner herself, the ability of our being able to discern what lies behind the question and our own competence to avoid platitudes. The spiritual impulse is to assist the questioner, the person in crisis, to discern the meaning inherent in that crisis. The comfort is in being there for the other. We all need a friend.

Doyle (1992) reiterates the perspective of identity as it is related to social relationship. In his experience of working with terminally ill patients he found that not only are they challenged by a new identity of 'dying' or 'disabled' but also about being needed. One of the expectations of legitimately achieving the status 'sick' is that we are no longer able to carry out our social obligations. Yet it is those social duties that lend many of us our identities. People fear that if they are of no further use socially then they will be disposed of. We see this in the enhanced rates of suicide among the elderly (Aldridge 1998).

Religion and public health

Religion and medicine have united to provide welfare programmes and fostered the establishment of community health programmes for education, screening and prevention (Chatters, Levin and Ellison 1998). While such programmes are not directly involved in curing illness, they offer a means by which the poor and disaffected can gain access to health-care delivery. Where residence in a poor community is a determinant of mortality and living in a deteriorating neighbourhood brings adverse health effects, then access to religious communities may have a beneficial influence by providing a sense of social integration and, pragmatically, by offering health-care programmes.

Krause (1998) surveyed a broad group of elderly people (mean age of 73.8 years old at the time of the initial survey). His initial hypotheses are that elderly people living in a dilapidated environment experience physical health problems more than older adults living in a better neighbourhood, and that such deleterious effects would be ameliorated by religious coping responses.

His findings are that older adults do indeed have more problems, the worse the living conditions become. However, religious coping brought no improvement in functional disability as an outcome measure. There is an improvement in the self-rating of health. People feel better through their faith. Self-rating is a global rating of how the person evaluates their own health at the time as excellent, good, fair or poor; how they are satisfied with their health and how they experience their health in comparison to others. Functional disability is concerned with concrete daily activities like climbing a flight of stairs, grasping a handle, carrying heavy bags, dressing, feeding and doing household chores. Religious coping may help people feel better, but there were no significant advantages in what they could do.

Carers as well as receivers

Religious coping in terms of prayer, bible reading, singing and worship, when it appears in groups, brings people together in times of adversity. It seems reasonable to suppose that this will improve the way that people feel about themselves. Traditionally religion has been seen to provide cohesion at times of fragmentation. Not only is there the chance for individual emotional expression within a caring group, but those expressions are brought to the attention of potential caring agencies. For welfare to achieve its aims, it must be aware of the needy. Church groups have functioned in the broader aspect of community health care to provide a means for the expression of distress.

Expressing a need and coping is only one part of the solution. What the expression of need achieves is the delivery of welfare and the delivery of welfare, as charity, benefits the giver as well as the receiver. Most major religions have a central component of compassion. The Other is to be recognized and served. It is this mutuality of the needy and the provider that is important for understanding health programmes in religious communities. Outcomes based on what happens to the receivers will always be one-sided. Future research will need to consider both receivers and providers, for here is the axis of mutuality that characterizes religious community life. If we talk about a performed health care, then it is the performance of the carers that is as vital as the performance of the receivers in determining the health of communities.

The construction of identity as sanctuary in crisis

Meanings are actively constructed. A personal approach structures how events are construed for the individual. We make sense of our lives. When our construings of the world are not recognized by others, when the way we see the world fails to be validated by others, then we have a situation where we face becoming increasingly isolated or we change those construings in accordance with how others see the world. This is the social element of construing the world. Among such social construings that we share are those cultural understandings which we call 'religious' and they are concerned with a relationship to the sacred. Our understandings of the world and those of others are discerned by what we do. Mutual understandings are negotiated in interaction with each other and these interactions themselves are made appropriate within a cultural context.

Religious groups offer a safe haven for such interaction. When identities are being challenged by crises, then a group of people with a set of recognizable beliefs and practices is a traditional means of providing stability for the threatened person. Such groups, however, are also purveyors of meanings and the activities by which meaning can be made. Rather than seeing a solipsistic world of individualized meaning, I am proposing that we make meanings from the stuff which we are offered to make meanings with. These are available within cultures. That is what culture does; it offers meanings and ways of discovering meaning. Thus meanings are not solely individual, leaving us isolated, but shared. Creatively, we can generate new meanings and offer them up to the cultures in which we live. This is how cultures remain lively by extending the totality of meanings and practices that are available. Cultures are enlivened when new initiatives are made. However, cultures are conservative. Meanings are conserved by groups and may be threatened by perceived change and the erosion of values when new understandings are not satisfactorily negotiated. The culture of healing has been enlivened by the debate of complementary medicines and the need for a reconciliation of religion with health. While there has been resistance from entrenched cultures of protective professional practice, these are being eroded by a broader culture of health-care delivery as influenced by the consumer who is seeking meaning and purpose.

A safe haven in crisis

Providing a safe haven for those in crisis is an activity of many religious organizations. This is the provision of sanctuary and refers to both a place that is inviolable and a holy place to the sacred. Park (1998) studied two religious congregations offering sanctuary for refugees. She too sees the religious as elevating the profane to the scared. What can be seen as an activity in purely social terms takes on a sacred meaning for those involved apart from the instrumentality and rationality of the profane world (p.408). People felt 'called' to act.

What marks these actions of sanctuary is that they are actions prohibited by US law. Actions by various church communities were in defiance of governmental decree. To participate is to be involved in breaking the law with the potential cost of arrest and heavy fines. Thus, the profane act of offering shelter is elevated to a sacred activity by religious meanings that are attributed by the congregations involved. By defying the threat of punishment, it is possible to demonstrate a commitment to values other than the material. In these instances, the sacrifice of material benefits is seen by the participants as increasing the validity of religious principles. Those taking part could claim a moral identity based upon their religious beliefs that is demonstrated in action. This identity is then further legitimated by the community of believers. Some religious groups will be composed of members who are seeking a moral identity, where sacrifice confirms the legitimacy of beliefs and actions.

In the suicide book (Aldridge 1998), it was exactly this construing of activity on a hospital ward and the legitimization of mutual meanings and behaviours that led to either a resolution or escalation of distress. The Weberian perspective on religion is just this. Religious belief formulates standards for behaviour and a politic regarding the implementation of such behaviour; how people behave, the meanings they have about what they do, and what they do is a political activity. The use of 'political' here is with a small 'p' referring to when individuals or groups cajole or seek to influence another group about how to act and how reality should be interpreted. We see this in the regulation of emotions and the forms that those emotions take.

What is salutary from this work is that the benefit of sanctuary is not only for those receiving sanctuary but also for those providing sanctuary. We may also say the same of some religious groups providing healing initiatives. The benefits are for the recipients and the providers. For the providers, the so-called healers, it demonstrates a commitment to beliefs, sometimes through material sacrifice, that also offers a moral identity. In modern health-care delivery we also see the emergence of self-help groups and groups interested in health promotion outside the professional health-care groups. The achievement of health is seen not only as an activity for patients but a communal activity that integrates both users and providers. Indeed, it is in the integrative activity, where 'provider' and 'user' are redundant concepts, where healing is taking place. While we may separate healer as doctor and healee as patient for the terms of understanding health-care outcomes in a scientific medical sense, in religious healing and other health-care initiatives it is the common activity that contributes to health in a community.

Religion as ligature

Religious practices are concerned with dietary observances, prayer consider-ations, the circumstances surrounding devotions, the receiving of sacraments and the recognition of holy days. In the separation of spirituality and religion then we have the current condition where religious practices through their moral identities are also used to separate groups of people. Most modern wars are based on ethnic conflicts related to religion. At a time when spirituality is concerning itself with private meaning and a search for unity, we have the opposite situation of public demands for ethnic identity based on religion and a demand for autonomy. Rather than there being practices that lead to a fullness of life we are seeing the decadence of religious observance that invalidates or annihilates the Other.

While it is necessary to respect the religious beliefs of patients and providers (and as we shall see later in Chapter 6 this is not without conflict), religion without its spiritual dimension is dangerous. The traditional purpose of religion was to offer a structured approach to the seeker through differing stages in which unity with the divine could be achieved (Shah 1990). Once religion loses this teaching approach, it runs the danger of becoming a political activity based on moral identities, or those of ethnic separation. Indeed, the Latin word *religare* is used as the source of the term religion meaning 'to bind' (Sims 1994), like a ligature, to a set of beliefs as a creed. When this happens, and a spiritual understanding that searches for unity and tolerance is abandoned, then we have the grounds for conditioning, a corrupted faith. Thus the brutalities of religious fundamentalism arise when the life blood of spirituality is prevented from achieving its goal. The ligature element of religion prevents such a flow. We also see a similar metaphor in ancient healing traditions that emphasized the flow of blood as the conveyor of life-giving spirit, or the flux of energies and humours. Once religion restricts the experience of the spiritual, then the flow of vitality ceases.

Religion is also integrative by intent and offers a set of meanings by which the flux of daily life can be understood. These sanctified meanings have a moral authority that is arbitrated by a priestly class. This is the function of ideology. The attribution of meaning through religious practice establishes the legitimization of social authority for actions. This also extends the political function we saw in the previous section to a community basis. Religion offers a critique of various systems of power, while maintaining a singular authority of power itself. We see this in the emergence of orthodox religious groupings playing an increasing political role in former communist countries and as the basis for escalating ethnic conflict. It has been the basis for an overthrowing of governments in the Near East and has been the crux of the conflict in Northern Ireland. Religious wars throughout history were never spiritual in their aims, but were expressions of nationalist loyalties and challenges for power. Indeed, nationalist rhetoric will often take on the symbols and emotions of religion in the name of salvation for a whole community (Cupitt 1997; Riis 1998). What unites them is that they are both examples of ideology.

In the same way we have an exercise of power in which medicine imposes an ideology of what it is to be sick and how that sickness is to be managed; how it is to be understood through research and how it is to be regulated through clinical practices and health-care delivery. This is no new phenomenon. Medicine has always had an ideological function and is based on a moral reasoning about the proper regulation of the body, how that body may be constituted – remembering that now we have the direct potential for genetic engineering – and how death may be regulated. There is a political element to the definition of subjective freedom as it concerns the body that the medical discourse attempts to define as scientific, as if it were not an ideology (Alter 1996). Alternative medicines are not free from this ideological aspect and it is on these grounds of biomorality that they are criticized by conventional medicine. On a public health scale, there is an ideological demand that we think in terms of population rather than individual meanings or personal localized relationships (Alter 1997). It is a rejection of such ideologies that has led to the emergence of new religious movements and alternative spiritualities.

Religious coping and the transcendent

Ideologies and their propagation through institutions are also seen as being positive in that they bind human beings to a stable set of ideas. This has been the stability argument, that we are protected from our own reckless and destructive nature. However, in modern societies there is a tension between institutions and personal freedom. Somehow that very tension has become institutionalized. Individuals are consumed by the institutions (Heidegren 1997).

Schelsky (Heidegren 1997) attempts to establish a critical distance to society with the notion of the *transcendental*, such that the freedom of the individual is to define the limits of the social. The individual is released from social causality and is, therefore, in a constant struggle with the institution. Each person will live out her autonomy through a 'way of life'. This way of living is not simply the interpretation that establishes meaning but is a performance of specific actions. Performance transcends knowing. From this perspective we have the notion of lifestyle that will come to the fore in the next chapter. Both a religious identity and health are experienced as performed realities encompassing a broad spectrum of daily practices. Thus we have performed identities, where becoming 'healthy' is a mixture of the religious and spiritual based upon a praxis aesthetic.

Riis (1998) sees religion re-emerging as a moral protest against political elites, as we saw in the sanctuary example above. This is not a return to the past. Secularization is an ideology that supports a particular power structure and tries to insulate a political elite from moral critique. Religion, as a world view, has the possibility of withholding or granting legitimacy to systems of power. This occurs at critical moments of life or death, in debates concerning the sanctity of life and means of reproduction, about the expression of sexuality and the maintenance of identity – as in the current development of genetic technologies. Where secular science attempts to discuss these matters, as if there were no moral responsibility, religion then assumes the role of an moral arbitrator. The same can be said in the delivery of health care when it threatens to lose its universality of delivery. Where the needy are granted a poorer service than the better off, then religion provides not only immediate welfare and a community of compassion but can also act as moral arbitrator.

The ethics of caring

Women appear to be more religious than men in Western societies and have turned to churches for social and emotional support when times are hard (Walter and Davie 1998). As we have seen earlier, a community of believers can provide compensations for a deteriorating city life. Despite immense developments in medical technology, there is still a need for a contact with the sacred at times of sickness, birth and death. What religions offer at these times are narratives related to such events that raise them beyond the instrumentality of technological circumstance to sacred moments. While medicine strips such occurrences to the routine procedures of daily life, instrumentalizing those processes to necessary sterile and efficient procedures, religion restores a sense of awe and wonder to living as a vitality of experience. It is not the birth or the death itself that is important, but the episodes of caring. As we have seen earlier with the giving of charity and the offering of sanctuary, both giver and receiver are united in the mutuality of care. In these moments, there is the possibility of transcendence to be realized. This is the unification of the element of transcendence that is essential to spirituality and its manifestation in daily life as the religious. The symbolic is restored.

Religious communities offer narratives of caring that elevate women's experiences from the instrumental to the divine. This was the original impulse of welfare as the basis of compassion, to treat the Other as yourself. At birth, we experience both the vulnerability and dependency of the young. This also raises issues for men. In a secularized society based on competition, power and ambition, recognizing vulnerability promotes an ethic of connection that produces the ethic of care. Now that birth has become safer in Western societies, through raised public health standards, and palliative care for the dying is becoming acceptable, there appears to be a renaissance of spiritual concerns in medicine, as we saw in Chapter 2, that meets our needs for a rich symbolic life.

Earth and its healing

These spiritual concerns are being psychologized and co-opted by a medical rationalization (Walter and Davie 1998). We begin to see a quantification of that care and attempts at an instrumentalization of spiritual healing. As a result of this attempt to quantify care and limit the possible explanation by operationalization, then we also see a postmodern spirituality emerging that involves the sacrilization of nature as earth religions and paganism. These movements are often female in structure and leadership having the individual as the ultimate authority, rather than a church-controlled authority with a male priestly hierarchy. This has led to the critique that they are anti-rational. Authoritative dogma is denied and replaced by an individual seeker of experiences, the praxis aesthetic referred to earlier. It reflects a similar movement in health care where dogmatic authorities are rejected and the individual seeks his own identity as 'healthy'. This identity is performed in varying contexts where it gains validity and recognition, but these contexts are temporary and there is an underlying ethic of care that is relational. Not so much 'I think, therefore I am', but 'I relate, therefore I am', or 'I relate, therefore we are'.

A return to a so-called spirituality of the earth has produced alternative or counter-cultural communities (Bloch 1998). These are not highly organized religious communities and probably favour the term spiritual rather than religious. At the core is a sought absence of dogma and social control. It is this dislike of dogma, the rejection of 'God said' and the idea of a counter-culture, that gives these individuals a sense of commonality, and thereby a collective identity. Heresy becomes taken for granted. The religious quest becomes a lifestyle preference and sensation seeking is part of the motivation in what Streib (1999) calls 'Off-road religion'.

Alternative religions argue that all aspects of life are sacred. Trees, mountains, rivers and all natural formations are seen to possess an animating force or spirit (Bird-David 1999). Saving the earth by promoting natural cycles of growth and improving the environment is potentially a spiritual activity. This is not necessarily a flight from science since scientific theories of ecology are used as foundational arguments in a rejection of the dogmatism of fundamentalism, whether that fundamentalism be religious or scientific. We have a bricolage of scientific rationality and spiritual thinking that attempts to build individualized world views adaptable to environmental goals, something like a survival spirituality that sounds like a sacred ecology. If the earth is seen as separate from the sacred, then there is an inherent dualism. Indeed, the fight against dualism has become the new dogma of the anti-dogmatic. In the flight from dualism we have the opposition of the alternative religions to the mainstream. The same goes for the identification of a female spirituality that emphasizes relationship and no hierarchy as opposed to male institutionalized religious affiliations (Rodriguez 1999).

With such challenges to authority, we have to consider religion in a post-denominational age. While the strength of denominational religion is that it offers a community joined by a set of shared meanings achieved through prescribed practices, we now see an inflation of the individual who joins with others in a common cause which is the maintenance of his own integrity. Where there was a sacred canopy that covered a variety of public religious expressions, we now have a camp of the individualized tepees of the new religious movements. The individual sets the terms for what is needed and chooses the forms required to satisfy those needs. Institutionalized forms may be adopted or abandoned to satisfy those needs. The same could just as easily be said of the health-care environment.

The conditions of modern life

New religious movements are concerned with secularization and the conditions of modern life (Dawson 1998). Some protest about changes in the pattern of social life and its ensuing alienation. People are searching for new structures of meaning and these give rise to new religions. Such religions can be seen as successor movements to the political protests of the 1960s and 1970s in that they are counter-cultural.

From another perspective, established religions are perceived as lacking in that they have become worldly and meet a demand for a relevance which is material and temporary. Individuals are left with a sense of yearning for moral guidance in an alienating culture, seeking a sense of self that is more than the limited functional roles that they are offered. With the rationalization of religions, and indeed health-care practices, then we see a loss of the latent social functions that bring cohesion. Religious and health-care traditions must adapt to the realities of privatization and pluralism, to a world where ideas, beliefs and practices are marketed. In advanced capitalist societies we are concerned with health care as 'commodity'. The same goes for religious identities such that they become entwined in a 'mix and match' pastiche of the individual in society.

With globalization we see a recognition of identities that go beyond former boundaries of family, village or community. We see young people wearing similar clothes, eating similar foods and enjoying similar music on a global scale. The influence of religion on diet, dress and behaviour has waned. Identities are being shaped by an interactive order that is electronic through communication media that are not immediately local, like the web. With this globalization we are seeing a corresponding demand for 'expressive individualism'. Each person wants to fashion and maintain a personal identity that is attractive and unique. We see people striving to achieve identities that relate to this global matrix, not necessarily to a communal group or local church. Identities are literally fashioned individually from a global market of offerings. New religious frameworks offer a vehicle for transcending a social identity that is based on given roles and a set of revitalized meanings by which the world may be understood. From this perspective, the web of a dispersed electronic community or even a broad ecological concept such as 'nature' are used as the societal matrix from which understandings are generated.

Coda

Religious activities offer ways of externalizing and perceiving the sacred. There are social practices in faith communities that promote meanings by which daily life and its contingencies may be understood and transcended. Transformation of the self is seen as a legitimate purpose of healing (McGuire 1996), but from a Durkheimian perspective this would be to achieve a social self, promote communication and achieve cohesion. Human suffering and distress are relieved by promoting a symbolic understanding beyond the instrumental interventions of scientific medicine. This is not a rejection of scientific medicine but an acknowledgement of its limitation, just as an understanding of symbolic meanings alone, without intervention, would be inadequate. Understandings have to be enabled and it is through faith communities that the necessary practices for enabling understanding can be achieved. The structure of such faith communities has traditionally been as 'churches', but these are now being challenged by new religious movements.

Similarly for health-care, there is a move towards health-care practices that are not simply based on conventional delivery in the sense of an authoritative, hierarchical practitioner administered medicine, but on consumer informed lay initiatives. However, if Durkheim's hypothesis that social action, like religious practice, promotes feelings in the individual of a moral force that is the basis of human understanding, then we have to consider the implications of increasing individualization and the restriction of social activity through electronic media. While we may be able to share data throughout the world, we have to ask ourselves where are we going to promote those elements of social cohesion through social action if people do not gather together. Social action, as inter-course, is a form of communication that is qualitatively different from the sharing of electronic data through a network displayed on a computer screen.

When we consider the continuing prevalence of suicidal behaviour in the young and the old, then they have become isolated from social interaction. The moral forces that have to be maintained to keep us alive and healthy are lost from daily practice as intercourse. Action is necessary for a sense of meaning, and action and meanings are important for health. Religion, as delivered through religious groups, has been one way of acting with a social purpose to provide and maintain health. The concept of 'health' I am using here is at a fundamental level of human living, not simply as a cultural expression of health-care delivery, and more akin to Durkheim's moral force.

One of the difficulties of the Internet is that people are separated from each other physically. Sensuality is marginalized. Science mistrusts the sense, pref-erring the regulation of machine data. In place of this we have the possibilities of sensual stimulation by machines in terms of virtual reality. Realities can be constructed without any human sensual contact. This effectively removes a significant scope of human learning and the potential for transcendence. Sim-ilarly, we see people meeting together as crowds to satisfy a human need for warmth, but with the express purpose of entertainment or to demonstrate in protest. These meetings are predominantly with temporary purposes and with limited expressive capabilities. Destructive barbarism is a real threat in modern societies and when we wonder what the sources are perhaps we may need to address the poverty of the social opportunities that we offer while we are commercially exploiting the advantages of the Internet. If we become indifferent to our neighbours and do not even see them, let alone speak to them, then we open up the morally vacant spaces of narcissism.

Healing and religion

Religious healing, while attempting to incorporate itself into modern health-care delivery, has also been a dissident religious movement challenging the authority of the churches (Aldridge 1986; Finkler 1994). However, both conformity and deviance demonstrate commitment to a common community. Science supports modern health-care delivery, but it is a sacred reality to which spiritual and religious initiatives turn. When a person seeks help to relieve his distress, then pragmatism prevails. We may use both the sacred and the profane in repertoires of healing. What religious healing attempts is to transform the situation in which a person lives. While this transformation has become indirectly social through welfare and advocacy within a socio-political system, the original impulse was social and directly aimed at changing consciousness through ritual. New understandings were gleaned through the social. Meanings were transcended through religious practice; the spiritual was attained. This is the change in consciousness we saw that was part of the spiritual intent described in Chapter 2. While the medical practitioner is concerned with the necessary biological changes associated with disease, it is changes of consciousness embodied in the social that bring about health. The concept of embodiment and health will be the topic of the next chapter.

The social is what is common to all religions. It offers forms for experiencing nature and the divine for transforming the self that is the goal of human development. Consciousness, achieving truth, is a social activity dependent upon its embodiment in individuals. Culture is the specific manifestation of such social forms in symbols, language and ritual localized for temporal and geographical contexts, thus specific cults and cultures. In globalization we have the dissemination of culture but without social forms related to human contact. I use the word dissemination advisedly here, as the global spread of ideas is like a rampant male ejaculation, intent on spreading its offspring wherever possible. The feminine aspect of relation and containment is relegated to the background. We have a masculine technology for the scattering of ideas, but we have not developed the feminine aspect of relationship by which those ideas can be contained and grown to maturity. This is literally the dissemination of data that fails to become in-form-ation. How to bring data into form and then apply that information is central to the development of human culture. If we fail to offer form through social intent then we will simply partake in a cultural onanism on a massive scale.

4

Lifestyle, charismatic ideology and a praxis aesthetic

A pure aesthetic expresses, in rationalized form, the ethos of a cultured elite or, in other words, of the dominated fraction of the dominant class. As such, it is a misrecognized social relationship. 'The denial of lower, coarse, vulgar, venal, servile – in a word, natural – enjoyment, which constitute the sacred sphere of culture, implies an affirmation of the superiority of those who can be satisfied with the sublimated, refined, disinterested, gratitious, distinguished pleasures forever closed to the profane. That is why art and cultural consumption are predisposed, consciously, and deliberately or not, to fulfil a social function of legitimating social differences. (Randal Johnson quoting Pierre Bourdieu 1993)

What is important is not liberation from the body but liberation from the mind. We are not entangled in our own body but entangled in our own mind. (Thomas Merton 1998)

The sources for this chapter are incidents taken from daily life. These incidents indicate the difficulties that we face when we talk about health and the practices that are used to maintain and promote such health. Indeed, one of the significant points of this chapter will be that health is heterogeneous and that such ideas come out of the practice of daily living rather than being homogeneous and based upon a rationalist unified theory. Such a demand for rational consistency may be misleading (Kirmayer 1993) and hide the discrepancies between varying forms of knowledge. This is not to say that we do not have coherent understandings of what it means to become ill, the process of recovery and the nature of distress and its relief which we can share with others, simply that there is a slippage between those understandings and the network of symbols which we have. These understandings of becoming ill and regaining health are not fixed like a set of natural laws although they may appear to follow local and temporary rules (Aldridge 1998).

While the above Bourdieu quote is made with regard to art and literature as cultural processes, the ascription of sickness and the meanings surrounding healing are also cultural processes (Csordas 1983, 1997; Fabrega 1997; Kleinman 1973a, 1978). Similarly, a refinement of arguments about the sacred nature of healing, as opposed to the profane nature of the vulgar body, legitimizes the availability of some healing endeavours to a particular class of consumers with the wherewithal to purchase those more sublime services.

Spiritual and religious healing, when referred to as a complementary medical approach, may appear to be confined to a particular well-heeled consumer group. However, as a traditional or folk medicine throughout Europe, such healing has sometimes been the only approach available to the poor where other medicines have been unavailable (Lewith and Aldridge 1991). Non-availability of these health-care initiatives may be made on grounds of cost, but what we have to remember is that in many rural areas the availability of health-care delivery is also dependent upon how health and illness are understood by the local population. While in Western industrialized nations we take a public high technology medicine with university trained practitioners for granted, there are many regions in the world where the consumers and deliverers of health care are differently educated and where a differing set of meanings is applied. In these regions unavailability of a medicine may be on grounds of education and culture and may refer directly to the domestic, rather than the public, domain (Stacey 1991). Furthermore, within the midst of the affluent nations and a triumph capitalism, we still have the poor, the elderly and the needy. How we respond to their needs is a measure of our civilization. This is not a technological response but a moral imperative.

Health as identity

In modern times, health is no longer a state of not being sick. Individuals are choosing to become healthy and, in some cases, declare themselves as pursuing the activity of being well. This change, from attributing the status 'being sick' to engaging in the activity of 'becoming well', is a reflection of a modern trend whereby individuals are taking the definition of themselves into their own hands rather than relying upon an identity being imposed by another. Being recognized as a 'healthy' person is, for some, an important feature of a modern identity. While personal active involvement has always been present in health-care maintenance and prevention, a new development appears to be that of being a 'healthy', 'creative', or 'spiritual' person. Such factors are considered to be significant in the composition of an individual's 'lifestyle'. Rather than strategies of personal health management in response to sickness, we see an *assemblage* of activities designed to promote health. These activities are incorporated under the rubric of 'lifestyle' and sometimes refer to the pursuit of 'emotional well-being' (Furnham and

Boughton 1995). Furthermore, such a lifestyle is intimately bound up with how a person chooses to define him or herself.

Modern identities are constructed. Although these identities are bound up with cultural values, they focus primarily on the body. What we need to take heed of as health-care professionals is that this 'body work', this embodiment of culture (Kirmayer 1993; Lowell Lewis 1995; Starrett 1995; Turner 1995), this corporeality of expression, is a pleasurable activity, often recreational and simply not medical. Bodies are performed. They become the material aspect of both the individual and the culture in which he or she is embodied.

By concentrating on the modern sense of self, there is a continuing focus on the body. Our corporeality is both objectified and subjectified, in that the body has become the major site of subjectivity and agency (Waterhouse 1993). When identity is constructed and traditional values, like gender, are challenged, there are times when individuals seek to establish identities that can be variously interpreted. White and Gillett (1994) illustrate this in terms of the muscular physiques of bodybuilders as a reaction to the erosion of power felt by men in the face of emancipatory forces that seek to challenge the ideology of gender difference.

'Bodywork', a term that occurs in numerous complementary medical approaches, locates cultural disciplines within a particular site, the body. The body becomes a commodity. It is seen as natural and culturally desirable and is developed through techniques (diet and training) and display. Malson (1999) refers to this as body-as-image rather than body-as-body. The individual is linked to the social. Feeling naturally superior, with a muscular self-made body, brings a link with social desirability and thereby coherence and meaning. However, this identification, within a plurality of cultural identifications, is offensive to others who are not masculine, or indeed, those who are not so muscular. Furthermore, as White and Gillett (1994) argue: 'Because real-power is located in economic and political structures, bodybuilding constrains the construction of identity to the pursuit of self-as-commodity. And, ironically, the elusiveness of the muscular ideal makes the self-transformation process ... a self-disciplinary dream rather than a lived reality' (p.35). But if White and Gillett's muscular body attempts an identity that is illusory, we also have the opposite extreme in Malson's (1999) anorexic body where identity becomes elusive in a material form that disappears. Both use body as image, as presentation that fails to satisfy the lived experienced body as it is. If thinness is socially desirable, as evident control over the passions and urges of the body, then this is offensive to those who are not so feminine, or indeed those who are not so thin.

Individuals seek to make identity claims in interaction within the context of culture. Claiming to be a spiritual person, or to be a 'spiritual healer', is a way of presenting self that will elicit a response from others. Corporeality, as presentation, has become spirituality. The circle has closed upon itself. Body and soul in modern descriptions are indeed united. Yet the soul, becoming incarnate in a postmodern body, is in danger of losing touch with the divine. How we maintain such souls intact depends on the dynamic interplay governing the transaction of all commodities, symbolic worth, market value, cultural need and spiritual emergency.

Catching a cold is your own fault

I caught a cold recently. Not that I went out one wet dark night, grabbed a cold and brought it home with me like an angler catches fish. Yet, in talking about this cold, which at times became *my* cold, I used a particular description common to our culture which most people understood, which few people questioned and which had little to do with the process of infection. This is not an isolated example. We still talk about the sun rising and setting as if the sun orbited the earth, yet we know theoretically and experientially that the earth orbits the sun.

In addition, I had this cold as an object like most of us have refrigerators. While we know that a cold is a process of infection and recovery, it actually achieves the status of an object. Hence it can be caught and got rid of.

My first inklings that something was different followed a weekend decorating the kitchen at home. Not only was I tired, but I developed a sore throat. I mentioned this soreness to my wife who concluded, quite rightly, that I had had enough of decorating; and, quite wrongly, that the soreness in my throat was a result of 'dust'. My mother, too, in a later telephone conversation, proposed that soreness must be a result of the dust produced in the process of decorating our apartment. This illustrates an interesting theoretical point. In making sense of a situation and in particular 'symptoms', causation is attributed to an agent, i.e. dust, in the context of a temporal event, i.e. decorating.

Later that same day things had taken a turn for the worse. My nose began to run. Given this information my mother's diagnosis would have been quite different. In my family of origin 'colds' are caught as a direct result of negligence. Either one goes out too soon after having a bath, neglects to wear a vest or discards clothing too early in the season. This has recently been tempered by an acceptance that living in centrally heated conditions is bad for you, especially if one goes from heat to cold. That is a sure-fire way of 'catching' a cold. There is certainly no notion of bacterial or viral infection. Catching a cold, then, was my own fault.

Infection, in my original family, is a term used by doctors and medical scientists which has no bearing on real life situations. Given the inability of modern medicine to cure the common cold, the notion of '*infection*' is of explanatory rather than practical value. Some concession is made to the notion of '*germs*'. These too, like colds, can be caught and exist in the ether like microscopic caterpillars or warm damp places which are not appropriate to be mentioned in a respectable book such as this.

By now the cold had definitely caught me. Like some monster it had invaded my whole being and quite literally had me by the 'throat'. After a night of fitful sleep my wife had changed her diagnosis to that of 'summer cold'. On arrival at work I received the first of a series of 'new' diagnoses. As my nose was well and truly recalcitrant to any air flow, the initial conditional diagnosis was that of 'hayfever'.

Hayfever and allergies are very big in our office with its emphasis on an holistic approach to medicine and psychoneuroimmunology. It is almost impossible to say psychoneuroimmunology with a head cold. The hayfever diagnosis went by the board quite quickly. Like all provisional hypotheses it was invalidated by further information. However, it did demonstrate an important part of the process of diagnosis. In lay terms the explanation of symptoms is initially dependent on a temporal context, i.e. a running nose in summer is likely to be hayfever.

Once I had croaked further details of the symptoms to my colleagues a firmer, more confident diagnosis was made. The basis for this diagnosis was made on observations of my general demeanour, the sound of my voice, the reported history I gave to my colleagues and the persistent use of tissues during the relating of this account. Thus, information in context aids the formulation of specific hypotheses.

A number of treatment suggestions followed this diagnosis. The principal injunction for treatment was to consume generous quantities of alcohol, notably whisky. To support this, what I assumed to be palliative, treatment I was encouraged to go home to bed. Presumably going to bed would avoid the iatrogenic problems of the treatment, i.e. falling down from too much alcohol. Not wishing to appear weak or sickly I struggled on at work.

A friend and colleague who is a general practitioner saw my plight, laid his hand upon my forehead and pronounced that I was feverish. Now that was the act of a true physician. I was soon to realize the personal and social implications of this viral infection. While willing to 'lay on hands' diagnostically, he refused to go out for a drink that evening when invited. Obviously the sick as persons are not to be mixed with and are temporarily not in the set labelled 'friends'. He suggested that I could meditate upon the meaning of the illness; yet another solution.

Another colleague, a woman of great resource, offered a more holistic comment on my plight. As a psychologist and psychotherapist in the 'humanist' tradition she broached the idea of stress, T-lymphocyte suppression and the possibility that this cold was occurring at a significant point in my life.

I must point out that during this process of escalating symptoms I had become irritable with friends and more and more despondent about the world in general and, as is usual at such times, was convinced that all my career decisions had been wrong. Those who favour a psychological approach to medicine will already be formulating a model which links depression, the suppression of T-lymphocytes, infection and physical symptoms. My perspective might be the other way round; cold (infection) first, depression later. However, as this is a chicken and egg situation, the best we can say is, and this is the point of the story, different explanations exist concurrently according to our own world views. The 'patient' does not always reflect the epistemological position of the observers.

One other consideration we may wish to make here is that when we talk of events we place them in a particular time frame. Events are, like this sentence, separated from other events by particular markers. Some theorists refer to this process as one of 'punctuation'. When we talk of episodes of illness we punctuate them by using certain markers from the general text of our lives.

First we note a difference. With my cold, you will recall, I first noticed that a sore throat and feelings of lassitude indicated a difference. In retrospect I could have perhaps detected other signs of an impending cold in the days before. To notice a difference then, we have to have some notion of threshold; i.e. when does soreness become sore enough to become noticeable? When does tiredness become lassitude? At the same time we attribute causality: Is tiredness a result of working hard or is it a symptom of infection?

In talking about this cold you will also notice that I am using a description of process. Symptoms escalate, albeit undetected, until they 'become' noticeable. The end of this process is marked by an absence of symptoms, although it seems that generally we have fewer markers for determining the end of a process than the beginning of a process. Stated in another way, I believe that we have developed a language which is refined in ways of talking about becoming ill, yet is impoverished in ways of talking about becoming well.

Meaning and implication: The semantics and politics of illness behaviour

When we talk about illness, whether it is taking the decision that we are 'ill' or making the decision to 'go home', which is a step in managing the illness, then we are making statements about our own beliefs and experiences in the world. The punctuation of an episode from the ceaseless stream of life's events has both semantic and political implications: semantic in the sense that explanations invoke meanings from a given episode; political in the sense that human behaviour is managed, obligations are suspended and actions are taken.

Both the semantic and the political are linked. Fay Fransella (Fransella and Frost 1977, p.24) writes: 'As a society we construct the social world according to our interests and beliefs, as individuals we construct our beliefs to make sense of our own particular experience of the world. So shared experiences and beliefs support each other – at least for a good deal of the time.' When we offer descriptions of our own behaviour to others, i.e. 'I have a really sore throat and I think I must have a cold', we are entering a realm where our description of a current reality is open to validation by another person. The validation of one person's description by another is a political act. While this may not have serious overtones in the context of a head cold, in that for me the only suspension of obligation was that I got out of doing the washing up for 48 hours, there are powerful implications for those who wish to have their experience of pain validated when it is not supported by physiological evidence.

In the context of a therapist–patient relationship, the patient offers up symptoms or descriptions which they believe entitle them to the legitimate status 'sick' (Parsons 1951). The therapist or doctor may interpret those same symptoms and descriptions as an example of the patient malingering and therefore making an illegitimate claim to the status 'sick'. In this context of consultation the therapist invalidates the patient, nothing is shared and a common legitimate reality is not negotiated (Aldridge 1998).

Life events

Life events have been seen as important precursors of illness. Mechanic (1974) points out the role that life events play in the occurrence of illness behaviour, but is careful to say that life changes, medical history, psychological distress and illness behaviour interact in complex ways. Although life events research has been predominantly oriented towards individuals and pathology, it also directs us to consider how individual life changes demand a complex response from the families of the individual (Dohrenwend and Dohrenwend 1974).

Within the literature there is a lack of consensus as to how individuals and families are influenced by life events, but the implication is that the way life events and life cycle changes are managed is crucial to health. We are left with a number of questions from the life events research:

1. How do some people and not others construe particular times and events in their lives as stressful (Folkins 1970; Hansen and Johnson 1979)?

2. How do some families collectively see some life events as indicators of change (Hansen and Hill 1964; Reiss 1981)?

3. How are some adaptations at the level of physiological functioning related to what people think and what their loved ones do (Lazarus 1974)?

4. What construings are resident within 'culture' that offer understandings of life events which attribute 'stress', and how do these affect individual

and family understandings (Mechanic 1966; Reiss and Oloveri 1983; Senay and Redlich 1968)?

Gregory Bateson (1972) offers an answer to these questions. He sees life events not as causative but as indicative. The recognition of a life event depends upon how individuals and social groups are informed by themselves and their culture as to what events make a difference. There is a process of co-evolution where individuals and social groups inform their culture and culture informs individuals and their groups (Aldridge 1998; Blumer 1972). Other researchers have described this relationship between culture and symptoms (Helman 1984; Kleinman 1978; Schwab and Schwab 1978) and cultural components in the expression of pain (Zborowski 1952; Zola 1966).

Eva, in Chapter 1, was trying to inform us that a loss of faith had caused her current plight. A faith had been 'lost' like a cold is 'caught'. Inherent in her causal description was the solution for recovery. No amount of medication was going to find her faith.

What counts as illness

If we take an episode of illness, which itself can be seen as a life event, then there are a number of stages in that episode when meanings are offered to others for validation. Making sense of the world is just that, a 'making' of sense. When we make sense it is made in the context of a relationship. Cecil Helman reminds us:

> Consultations between doctors and patients do not take place in a vacuum. Rather, they are embedded in a particular time and place, and in a particular physical, social or cultural setting. That is, each consultation is embedded in a particular context. These contexts are important, because they shape what is said in the consultation, how it is said, how it is interpreted, and how it is acted upon. (Helman 1986, p.37)

We can apply the same criteria of time and place to our personal relationships. Helman also goes on to distinguish internal and external contexts.

An internal context is the set of hidden assumptions and responses that each party brings to the relationship. These would include our past experiences of illness, the explanations for the origin of the illness and how symptoms should be treated. As we can see, 'my cold' was interpreted according to a number of internal contexts. It must be remembered that these contexts are not fixed but negotiated.

An external context includes the setting in which the event takes place as well as rules of conduct. In some ways an external context is a form of ritual. It is punctuated as being separate from 'everyday life' and governed by explicit and implicit rules of conduct about how people are to act, speak and dress and what they are to talk about.

At an obvious level we see this in public rituals like weddings, funerals and scientific conferences, but we also have ritualized ways of dealing with deference, greetings and leaving (Geertz 1957; Leach 1976; Vogt 1960).

At a more fundamental level we have our own internal rituals for recognizing 'stress' or 'no stress' that are based upon a highly complex immunological language which is more than a biochemical alphabet. This language can be used to identify what is 'self' and 'not self'. In such a way we are daily constituting ourselves. We make a sense of the world bodily. However, as we are all aware, we also make sense of the world psychologically, socially and spiritually.

Sometimes this bodily sense becomes evident in another realm of experience. When we experience pain then a message is being sent from one systemic level (somatic) to another (psychic). This message needs to be interpreted. It is not always immediately discernible what pain is a message about. For instance in the case of back pain is it about muscular distress, or is it a metaphor about distress in a different systemic context, for example, having too much to bear or a lack of support? In some recent research into the common cold (Aylwin, Durand and Wilson 1985) the researchers found that people with different representational styles (verbal, visual or enactive) had different ways of being ill. Verbalizers, people who use inner speech, were prone to mouth ulcers. However, visualizers showed no particular propensity for any problems but there was a negative correlation with relaxation and resistance to infection. Somehow literally the way we see the world and represent it to ourselves is a health enhancing activity. Making sense is not only a passive process, but an active process which we do to the world.

Rules for the making of sense

I suggested earlier that 'making sense' is rule based. A constitutive rule would be invoked when I say that this behaviour (a running nose) counts as evidence of another state (a cold). A regulative rule would be invoked when we say if this behaviour (a running nose) counts as evidence of a particular state (having a cold) then do a particular activity (go home to bed). Constitutive rules are generally concerned with meaning. Regulative rules are concerned with the politics of relationship and the linking of meaning and action.

The meaning of sickness and the control of healing functions are interrelated. Kleinman and Sung (1979) argue that modern professional health care attends solely to the control of sickness and neglects the understanding of meaning. Furthermore:

> The biomedical education of physicians and other modern health professionals, while providing them with the knowledge to control sickness, systematically blinds them to the second of these core clinical functions (the understanding of

meaning), which they learn neither to recognize or to treat. (Kleinman and Sung 1979, p.8)

If we return to the understanding of life events we could hypothesize that constitutive rules exist which identify particular acts as life events. Regulative rules would propose a way of handling such events.

In an episode of illness there will be stages when behaviour is understood in terms of constitution, that is meaning, and in turn, regulation, that is, control or management. Episodes have critical times when they are seen 'to start' and 'to end'. This is the process of 'punctuation' (Bateson 1978) and is a selective structuring of reality. Punctuation is vital to interaction as it is a means of organizing behavioural events both in terms of meaning and process.

We see this when Eva said that her problems began when her husband died. While such punctuations may be shared, they may also be the source of conflict. For instance, some of us may recall situations where one person has said, 'I was only trying to be helpful and support you' and their partner says, 'You were interfering and undermining my ability.' In such an exchange the two punctuations of the same behaviour helpful/interfering are a characterization of the relationship. This has been described as a 'rule' of the relationship (Aldridge 1998; Jackson 1965).

In our modern Western culture the predominant focus to punctuate the start of an episode of illness appears to be one of recognizing symptoms which are validated in the context of a relationship, whether it be familial, filial or fraternal. If we return to my sore throat we can see that in the relational context of marriage and family of origin and in the temporal context of decorating, a sore throat was seen as a result of dust and was not evidence of illness. The possibility of my having a cold was not validated.

However, after offering further evidence for validation, i.e. the classical symptoms of a cold and a fitful night's sleep, then I was recognized as having 'a cold'. My personal reality was negotiated and validated in the context of a relationship. Similarly as my symptoms persisted the various meanings inferred from them by others were used to offer a number of prescriptions for regulating that illness.

In terms of a cold this was quite straightforward as the causative agent was seen as a viral infection and not open to a great deal of debate and there was a general consensus of opinion that the only recourse was palliative. However, in considering other forms of illness meanings are not so clear cut, or can be perjorative.

Symptoms can be employed as a 'language' within a group of people (Kreitman, Smith and Eng-Seong 1969) and in particular families (Aldridge 1998; Haley 1980; Madanes 1981) where other groups would use less pathological forms of communication. Symptoms become part of a vocabulary of distress. As an example, pain would then become an indicator not only of physiological distress, but also a marker of existential despair, personal 'hurt' or unwillingness to co-operate.

We learn a set of shared meanings whereby symptoms located in particular contexts are understood in a particular way; i.e. the process of diagnosis. This corresponds to a set of 'constitutive rules'. Acupuncturists recognize disturbances in ch'i. Neurolinguistic programmers recognize maladaptive speech patterns. Structural family therapists see family coalitions and permeable boundaries. Transactional analysts hear 'the child' speaking in the adult. A priest recognizes the sinner and the sin. A spiritual healer discerns a loss or blocking of energy.

Similarly the process of diagnosis leads to implications for what to do about those symptoms, i.e. the process of treatment. This corresponds to a set of 'regulative rules'. The acupuncturist endeavours to restore balance. The neuro-linguist intervenes by talking directly to the somatic system responsible for the problem. The family therapist asks the family to change seats and move closer together. The transactional analyst encourages the adult to speak to the adult. The priest will confer absolution. The spiritual healer channels energy. God forgives. Here we have a significant shift. In spiritual and religious healing, the power has traditionally not been located in the healer, although this is now shifting with the move from traditional spiritual healing approaches to more eclectic methods where healers become 'empowered'.

The challenge for the therapist or practitioner is that although the symptoms reported by the patient may fit the practitioner's set of rule-based understandings, those rules and corresponding understandings may be quite different to those of the patient and the patient's family. All too often patient and therapist can be at odds because the important phase of negotiating common or shared meanings is missed out.

The implications for therapy are that we must be concerned with under-standing what the symptoms constitute for the patient and what the patient has previously done to regulate those symptoms. In a similar way, we must be aware that by the time a patient reaches the therapist or practitioner they have been through a process where their symptoms have been negotiated and validated in other contexts which may have far more significance for them as persons.

What I want to propose is that sometimes when we see people with persistent problems it may well be that their personal meaning system, their sets of constitutive and regulative rules, have been invalidated in other relational con-texts, and they too have invalidated the systems of meanings offered by significant others. When such a situation of mutual invalidation occurs and symptoms appear as 'intractable' then we find that the patient is given a label of deviance or described as rather resistant. Rarely do we hear that the therapist has failed to understand the patient. This too would be falling into a trap of blaming one person in the relationship rather than looking at the therapeutic process itself and the relationship between therapist and patient.

The process of deciding

Making and taking health-care decisions is a process. We become aware of events that make a difference. Some of these are seen as symptoms and as indicative of certain states. These constitutive rules are learned through experience and validated in the context of families and friends. We rarely have to invoke these rules as they are habitual. In the context of illness behaviour they form a repertoire for the management of distress (Aldridge 1998). Occasionally when we come into contact with other persons and other groups we find that those rules are questioned and that repertoire is inappropriate.

As these rules are learned in families they persist over time and can be carried over from one generation to the next. In this way some particular forms of illness behaviour such as depression appear to be hereditary. However, we have not as yet identified the genes responsible for depression and alcoholism. It could well be that neither depression nor alcoholism are hereditary but both run in families. At certain times and in particular situations, faced with personal failure in a context of relational conflict, there may be constitutive and regulative rules which propose particular behaviours, e.g. become depressed or drink to drown your troubles. These behaviours are learned in families and transmitted from one generation to the next, they become repertoires of distress management. If so, then they demand repertoires of distress relief that are systemic and not solely individual. Traditionally, religious healing has done just that by incorporating the patient or sinner within a healing community as we saw in Chapter 3.

Choosing to intervene

At which level then do we choose to intervene and at which point in the cycle do we choose to enter? A challenge for us as practitioners and researchers is to elicit those cyclic patterns of behaviour with their underlying rule structures whereby physiological changes occur in response to personal and relational crises. There may well be rules operating which say that in a specific context (an academic conference), a particular action (speaking to a group of one's peers) constitutes a threat and is to be regulated by a particular behaviour (elevated heart rate, increase in perspiration, suppression of lymphocytes). While this may well be 'normal' behaviour (and the attribution of normality itself is rule dependent), if there were a set of personal rules that interpreted all situations as threat (to be regulated by an elevated heart rate or a suppression of lymphocytes) then we might speculate that there is an underlying disease or at least a maladaptive coping strategy (Nixon *et al.* 1986).

In this sort of description diseases are not fixed or immutable. They are open to change at different levels of intervention; for example, a change in a constitutive rule would mean that some events would no longer count as crises; a change in a regulative rule would mean a change in response. We do this in treatment where some of us look for underlying attitudes and attempt to change them (the process of constitution), whereas some therapists will attempt to provoke changes in response to stimuli (the process of regulation).

This rule making is in a Jungian sense a problem of knowledge (Jung 1961).

> But what is recognition or knowledge in this sense? We speak of knowing something when we succeed in linking a new perception to an already established context in such a way that we hold in consciousness not only the new perception but this context as well. 'Knowing' is based, therefore, upon a conscious connection between psychic contents. (Jung 1961, p.112)

My argument is that these connections are rule based. It is important to remember the notion of rule is used here as a metaphor for what happens, not that there is literally a rulebook in the head or the family. The making of these connections is a change in consciousness which partially fulfils the definition of spirituality from Chapter 2.

Body as a source of consciousness

These rules need not necessarily be cognitive. They may act solely at the level of physiology where there are physiological changes occurring in response to biochemical markers in the context of immunological stress. As stated earlier, we need to address ourselves to the continuing problem of how the threat to a threshold at one level, i.e. the cognitive, brings about a response at another level, i.e. the physiological. A rules based explanation addresses this by offering a means of description (but not a causal link) of what happens. By understanding the interaction between these levels we can intervene at differing levels. We also see how the body is vital in the achievement of consciousness. Furthermore, we also see how changes in thought, behaviour and relationship have their ramifications for physiology and thereby the process of physical healing such that prayer (Byrd 1988; Dossey 1993; Koenig, Bearon and Dayringer 1989; Magaletta and Duckro 1996), laying on of hands (Benor 1990, 1992), therapeutic touch (Krieger 1979; Wirth 1993; Wirth and Cram 1997; Wirth et al. 1996b), and meditation can make a difference (Aldridge 1987b; Astin 1997; Kabat-Zinn 1993; Lukoff et al. 1998; Miller 1998b).

We must be aware that healers and patients are not independent of the cultural context of clinical care and the explanatory models we bring to bear on illness and healing are resident within this cultural context. In this way we will begin to understand the meaning of illness and the attendant implications for healing rather than the headlong pursuit into the management of disease. This changes clinical practice and research endeavours (Miller 1998b). A pluralistic tolerant system of health-care delivery will offer a variety of means for understanding problems as they are presented and, similarly, a spectrum of possibilities congruent with those understandings, such that those problems may be resolved.

However, we must be wary. The way we construct our meanings of problems, particularly when presented by the people who come to see us for therapy, may be a contribution to the way in which the problem is maintained rather than allowing change to happen.

Mind as unity

Bateson (1972, 1991) implies that in every unity, where there are conversation-like actions, there is an ecology of ideas and the presence of mind. Varela (1979) takes this notion further and talks about a mindlike activity beyond our own individual minds where there is a higher order of unity, which is not readily amenable to consciousness. Apart from sounding remarkably Jungian, it does point to a higher order of rules of constitution and regulation whereby we are made sense of and regulated. We are part of a system which accommodates us. We move from isolation (Hoffman 1985) to unity. As Varela (1979) writes:

> Thus we do not have…a world of shared regularities that we can alter at whim. In fact the understanding is beyond our will because the autonomy of the social and biological systems we are in goes beyond our skull, because our evolution makes us part of a social aggregate and a natural aggregate which have an autonomy compatible with but not reducible to our autonomy as biological individuals. (Varela 1979, p.276)

Defining health and the definers of health

The definition of health, who is to define what health is and who is to be involved in healing, is not a new activity. Such issues are raised at times of transformation when the old order is being challenged. As we read in Chapter 1, orthodoxies are challenged and truth is regarded as relative with few fixed authorities to turn to. Identities can be composed from a palette of cultural alternatives that are offered through a variety of social relationships.

Commodification

Health is also appearing in modern society as a commodity. Far from being a simple object, health is concerned with social relationships representing personal worth, market values, existential principles and theological niceties. However, the location of health in modern terms is often within the body (Charmaz 1995; Kelly and Field 1996; Wallulis 1994).

People are also demanding recognition that they play an active role in their own health-care, and that some can act as lay health-care practitioners. Indeed, before we ask a doctor or any licensed practitioner we have been through varying cycles of self-care, asking family and friends or just hoping that the problem will go away. This shift away from authority and orthodoxy towards democratization and choice reflects a change from a belief in the certainties of science and dogmas of religion to a relativist position where people talk as if they literally 'make up' their own minds and work on their bodies; that is, construct their own identities. From what has been written earlier in this chapter, a constructivist argument is not totally idiosyncratic. A palette of symbolic meanings and social relationships is simply extended and made available within social contexts. From a Durkheimian perspective, the social offers a repertoire of healing possibilities.

A government white paper in England (*Working for Patients*, January 1989) suggested a radical restructuring of health-care with emphasis on a consumer-based service. This reflects a growing movement throughout Europe whereby health-care initiatives are responding to consumer demand (Aldridge 1994). Some of these initiatives may be based on what is currently regarded as 'complementary' or 'alternative' medicine. A concerted European action (COST Action B4 Unconventional Medicine) recommends further an integration between conventional and unconventional approaches, that a common cure curriculum for acceptable training standards in health-care practitioners who are to be licensed by the state is established, and that appropriate constraints analysis for research are implemented.

This emphasis on consumer choice and demand reflects what happens anyway. People choose how they wish to maintain and promote their own health. A possible reason for the popularity of complementary medicine is that the involvement of the patient in his or her own health-care is recognized by the practitioner. Other reasons given for choosing complementary therapies are: that they may include a psychosocial approach to problems; that the patient's search for health is understood in terms of reasons and intentions; and that there is an acknowledgement of the intent of both parties to co-operate in health-care. There is less a turning away from orthodox medical care because of dissatisfaction, more a demand for mixed pluralistic health-care.

User needs predominate

In the patient's search for treatment formal health-care delivery often comes late in the chain of decision making. Only health professionals emphasize the formal health-care network, i.e. a 'top-down' approach. Health-care requirements in a consumer based approach are determined from the needs of the users, i.e. a 'bottom-up' approach. Health-care decision makers are also currently considering how health-care can be delivered in a pluralist European culture, i.e. one which acknowledges modern scientific, traditional and complementary medicine. A consumer based health plan, which emphasizes choice and includes alternative medicines, will be necessary to promote an atmosphere of permissive legislation for the control and licensing of a broad spectrum of practitioners and develop economic financing and delivery arrangements. The structure of such arrangements will depend upon knowledge of the process of health-care delivery and organization.

With these elements of individual choice and the secularization of what were once traditional spiritual disciplines, we find an emphasis on techniques of health-care that are available to both the lay public and to professional practitioners. This situation is perhaps best exemplified by the modern practice of meditation.

Secularization of meditation

Meditation has been the central plank of ancient spiritual disciplines, particularly those arising in the East. In the case of traditional Buddhist practices, meditation has played a significant role in the development of the novice as guided by the master. In almost all the traditions, both teacher and pupil, monk and novice, have been male and the content of the teaching has not been negotiated but firmly based on fixed disciplines of practice and embedded in ritual. Meditation, traditionally, has been located in a cultural context that has determined waking, sleeping, eating, posture, clothing and physical appearance.

In many modern Western alternative health-care initiatives, meditation has been removed from such a context of spiritual tradition and secularized. While some groups and individuals claim that they are 'spiritual' in that they use meditation, some forms of psychotherapy practice will use meditation as an example of a mind–body technique without any reference to spiritual practice.

As an example of the secularization of meditation, a book entitled *Mind Body Medicine* and subtitled *How to use your mind for better health* (Goleman and Gurin 1993), provides us with ample material. Of the thirty-three contributing authors, all but one are trained in medicine or psychology. The one eccentric author is a freelance writer concerned with health psychology and promotion. In the introductory chapter, in a section entitled 'What does it cost?', mind–body approaches are considered as generally inexpensive or even free: 'It costs next to nothing, for example, to learn the "relaxation response" – a basic method of meditation that is now used to treat a range of physical problems' (p.15). Here the physical benefits of an overtly psychological technique – further reduced to relaxation response – are married to the benefits of cost effectiveness. Similarly, the writer goes on to propose: 'And one reasonable alternative, among many, is to emphasise disease prevention by encouraging a healthy life-style – including mind/body methods – particularly for groups of people at risk for specific disease' (p.17). Disease prevention, while being taken from its former context of community health-care is both individualized and psychologized among an unspoken plurality of opportunities, while at the same time retaining the paradigm of modern scientific medicine that there are groups at risk for specific diseases.

In a later chapter elucidating the relaxation response (Benson 1993), this response is seen as a stress-reducing phenomenon regulating the 'physiological machinery' of the body. Originally part of a meditation technique, the biological response has been elevated to a central position, relegating the mind to an epiphenomenon and completely excluding any considerations of spiritual development or cultural relevance. The purpose of such beings are purely those of maintaining biological regularity in what is always potentially a challenging environment. It must be stated that the author of this chapter is Herbert Benson, a medical practitioner and professor of behavioural medicine, cited as an authority on relaxation and meditation, whose book about relaxation is still 'the self-help book most often prescribed by American psychologists' (Goleman and Gurin 1993).

When techniques of meditation are considered, then it is in support of the reduced response: 'Rather than practising transcendental meditation, individuals simply repeated the number one on each exhalation and passively disregarded any intrusive thoughts. As we predicted, we found changes that were indistinguishable from those of earlier findings with transcendental meditation' (Benson 1993). Prayer is also seen to be producing the same bodily response. It is recommended that religious patients use a prayer when they elicit the relaxation response or that non-religious patients use any sound or phrase with which they are comfortable. The idea that prayer may have a content or indeed a focus is nowhere discussed. That the relaxation response may be an even more powerful tool than the author can validate in his chapter is recounted in an anecdote concerning Tibetan Buddhist monks: 'In an annual ritual, these monks shed almost all of their clothes, wrap themselves in icy sheets on a near-freezing night, and proceed to enter a state of deep meditation...by doing this they are able to raise their skin temperature to levels warm enough to dry the sheets' (p.255). That this technique may not be an isolated incident and is itself part of a meaningful set of practices, other than self-laundry, is not even considered. Thus extreme control of the physical body is seen as a product of training the mind. The relaxation response, as a subset of meditation techniques, is used here rather like other 'body' mastery techniques such as body-building, exercise and dieting to gain, and presumably demonstrate, extreme control in the face of succumbing to that modern peril, stress. Indeed, the basic two-step practice includes the repetition of muscular activity and a passive return to that repetition whenever distracting thoughts recur is seen as a natural response and the opposite of stress. Human beings then, in their natural state, are seen from this perspective as a collection of physiological responses.

In the chapter immediately following, the health benefits of an ancient Buddhist practice are described (Kabat-Zinn 1993). While the emphasis is upon mindfulness meditation, the ultimate secular goal is that of stress reduction. Inner strengths are mobilized and behaviour changed in a new imaginative way over eight weeks. While mindfulness is admitted to be a complex discipline, the focus of the chapter is targeted upon the participants as patients and the purposes are those related to specific illness problems, as in the relief of chronic pain. 'Increased trust and oneness, along with other positive psychological changes' and 'a profound change in people's outlook on themselves in relationship to the world' are cited as benefits of this psychological approach. Furthermore, 'preliminary clinical studies suggest' (p.272), presumably with all the authority of an advertising campaign, that the mindfulness training programme can 'improve a range of physical symptoms; reduce pain; depression, and anxiety; enhance feelings of trust and connectedness; and help motivate patients to take better care of their health' (p.272). In a world where people are suffering, where they are isolated and demoralized, this plan appears to replicate the positive goals of the prayer groups suggested for the elderly in the black community, albeit expressed in different terms. The marginalized, sick and lonely are encouraged to join a group and motivated to take care of themselves. Identity is conferred by positive action.

However, as the chapter ends, we read that there is no commitment expected to a community of fellow believers, nor an acceptance of a taught doctrine, rather a singular commitment to self as lifestyle: 'Mindfulness meditation involves a significant commitment to oneself. More than a technique, it is really a way of life. Many of those who practice it find that it can deeply enhance their mental and physical well-being' (p.272). This approach reflects the liberal dilemma as seen reflected in the legitimacy claims of treatment approaches mentioned earlier; the romantic notion of the individual freedom, where individualism in terms of beliefs, desires and practices is emphasized at a time of social fragmentation and reorganization. However, what seems to be significant in the claims of spiritual healing is that while particular psychological techniques are borrowed from spiritual traditions, it is the body of the person that is chosen to express beliefs and desires through defined practices in the social realm.

Loss of orthodoxies

As a consequence of challenges to traditional authority and the collapse of state socialism in Europe, there is no longer a possibility for some individuals to relate to a given social order. Orthodoxies are described as dogmatic, restrictive and authoritarian. In the writings of many health-care practitioners, particularly in alternative medicine, there are few references to health-care as being a social product for the benefit of communities. Instead, rather than a communal discourse being voiced, there appears to be an argument for the individual located in an ecological context; the 'green' politic of environmental liberalism. Such a perspective ignores the notion of population and health and the pervading fact that morbidity is correlated with the distribution of wealth (Evans, Barer and Marmor 1994).

Individuals are seeking to treat themselves with a long-term eclectic health strategy that includes a palette of activities with the support of chosen, albeit diverse, informed advisers who can fulfil the role of facilitator. Health-care consumers are blurring the role between the traditional health-care services delivered at times of crisis with those of preventive strategies based on consumerism. The idea of community health in these descriptions may be alluded to as an ecological context, but there is little reference to an immediate social or communal context. This is a reflection of the Romantic notion of the individual related directly with the cosmos (Tsouyopoulos 1994), admittedly with like-minded others as a tribe of fellow travellers.

Talking about health

I am using illustrative anecdotes here for two reasons. First, through stories we see how health is a complex set of ideas. Second, as we read in Chapter 1, we need to consider the day-to-day narratives of individuals as they talk about health if we are to make sense of what health-care is appropriate as treatment and prevention. What I shall also be suggesting is that most research makes an assumption that health and illness are opposing poles of a continuum, which is a false premise. My proposal is that health and illness, as oppositional poles, may be so constructed by health-care professionals trained to think in such a way, but such an ideology may not be reflected in the everyday lives of other people. Perhaps the realms of health and illness are quite separate in practice? Rather than being oppositional they are competing arguments relevant for making sense of particular situations. This is not to reject medical explanations, rather to extend scope of what is permissible to make sense of illness.

Vulgar health

We saw earlier that being healthy is a process of validation and the legitimation of mutual understandings. Health is also a sensual activity.

At a meeting of anthropologists and health researchers in Denmark, following the usual presentations about health and various approaches to medicine, we duly retired to eat and then to the bar where several colleagues ordered their drinks and smoked cigarettes. For most of the day we had been sitting in a centrally heated room and had taken part in no strenuous activities other than disagreeing with each other in a mild sort of way and occasionally moving our chairs to let others get by. From some perspectives of health-care activity, we were behaving quite irresponsibly; smoking, drinking both coffee and alcohol, pursuing sedentary activities and, no doubt, eating fatty foods. However, those of us partaking in such activities seemed to be paying little attention to 'health' as such and were generally getting on with the day-to-day business of living, part of which was actively pleasurable. As such this is a rejection of an aesthetics of Kantian 'pure' taste and an embracing of a Bourdieuian 'vulgar' taste that returns to the senses. It is this notion of sense that is at the heart of the original meaning of aesthetic in that it springs from the lower animal passions, a matter of literal taste.

The next anecdote occurs in yet another country and is also concerned with health as pleasure but the inherent moralism of health-care. One of the joys, or burdens, of being a conference delegate is that one has to take part in social activities. It so happened that I was invited to the German beer festival in Munich and, not wanting to offend my hosts, I duly took part. The festival takes place in a huge park complete with fairground activities that are replete with noise and activity and charged with the electricity of human beings having fun. Within the festival grounds there are huge barns where people go to be entertained. The group I was with were duly led to such a barn and as the doors opened I was immediately reminded of many of the things my mother had told me not to do as a boy and which still seemed so enjoyable as a middle-aged man. From out of the open doors came a billow of smoke, gales of laughter, squalls of music from a German 'oompah' band and the wonderful breezy beery odours of the hall: all the perils of enjoyment captured together in a storm of experience. Like catching a cold was my own fault, it will be my own fault if I do not make it to old age.

Here lies the crux of the argument. Most of the health-care debates are moralistic and ignore a profound factor in human existence, repeated from the Danish conference example, and that is the importance of the simple activity of pleasure. These pleasures are perhaps temporary and rarely reflected upon for their health-care consequences, but they are vital in the broadest sense of the word. Thus we have a sense of sensual pleasure but a health-care mentality which emphasizes that it will probably be bad for us to enjoy ourselves. Religious admonitions similarly deny the pleasures of the body.

The flesh is weak

In the Christian tradition a perception of the body has been that the flesh is the source of temptation. As a consequence, pleasure is regarded as sinful. Bodies as a means of knowledge were ignored by the Christian communities, or such knowledge was considered to be evil (Van Ness 1999). The soul being imprisoned by the body was a Platonic concept. Being without the body was a preferred solution (Duvall 1998), albeit difficult to conceive.

When science and secular traditions took over from the Church as arbitrators of knowledge, then the body became a material entity and was lost as a site for a sacred arena in which a broader discourse of purpose could be elaborated. Little wonder then that postmodern understandings of a pleasurable body have seen a retreat from Christianity. New religions and health-care movements see the body as a site that can serve a positive purpose. This is perhaps why Eastern traditions of meditation and yoga have become attractive through the promise of body as a means of transcendence. Fitness and exercise, as health-care activities, have become part of an identity that is not simply material but which some consider to be religious (McGuire 1988, 1996) and are often linked to an identity that is deemed to be 'spiritual'. We have a return of the 'soul' in that body and mind are united as one inseparable entity.

Loss of tradition

If the self in modern society is always being constructed to meet the variety of life's contingencies, then we move away from the model of one generation initiating the next generation into the truths of its own beliefs. Instead there is a pool of experts and advisers to whom we can turn when constructing a system of beliefs within a cultural ecology; ecological, in the sense that those beliefs are connected and the consequences of those beliefs, when acted out in the real world, are related one to another. In some modern alternative healing approaches, traditional forms of teaching by initiation and learning by discipline are rejected in favour of an eclecticism that takes techniques and locates them within a culture of meanings improvised according to the situation. This action itself is political. Rejecting given orthodoxies and demanding freedom to engage in the project of realizing one's 'self' is a 'politics of life-decisions concerning life-styles' (Brewster Smith 1994). The rejection of tradition also means that oral traditions of healing are lost along with forms of initiation into practices of spiritual healing. There are some things that cannot be learned from books.

Health talk in a constellation of understandings

The third anecdote concerns talking about health as a part of social discourse. This scene occurred in a restaurant. My wife and I had decided to take an early spring walk. The weather was fine and after a gentle stroll we arrived at a hotel in time for lunch as planned. To my way of thinking, there is no point in a long walk unless you end it at a restaurant. Why waste all the exercise. During the meal, a number of middle-aged women came to sit at the next table. The first topic of conversation was their health and each woman took turns to talk about her current ailments. In doing so she introduced various connected topics like the state of her family, the well-being of her husband, the relative benefits of being mature, where she had been shopping recently for shoes and a general philosophy and outlook on life. While as professionals we might be tempted to look at this as a health-care narrative, health being the chosen topic of introduction, we would be missing a valuable point. Health was used as a springboard for a wide-ranging conversation that did not itself remain focused on health. Health-care issues provided a structure to the conversation as a recurring topic that punctuated the developing talk between the women.

Like the stereotypical greeting 'Hello, how are you?' rarely intends to elicit a conversation about the person's state of health, health as a subject of naturally occurring narratives plays a significant role but is not dominant. All too often we consider health as if it was the peak of a unified pyramid of rational consonant understandings, rather than a topic in a constellation of understandings, some of which may be dissonant. Knowing the relationships between elements of such a constellation might help us to understand health as part of daily living, as praxis. Health topics may act as a focus that organizes conversations between people when they talk from which the discussion can develop in varying directions. We can talk about our bodies, about our relationships, about our future, about our past, about our fears or about our potentials.

To make a complex matter even more complicated, we also have to remember that this story was set in a restaurant. Women were sitting together talking and eating. Their primary reason was social and that was organized around eating; not eating for its nutritional benefits but as a pleasurable experience. While their first topic of conversation may have been health, it was interleaved with a concurrent discussion related to the menu. Both topics converged on the dietary needs of the participants but these appeared to be cosmetic rather than clinical.

When we talk about health, we may use it as a general strategic structural topic to organize a conversation between friends and acquaintances. This is different to the structured conversation between patient and practitioner. Indeed, it is illness as a topic that may dominance the interaction. These are two different domains and only loosely related. To consider health as one end of a spectrum and illness at the other is an oversimplification.

The benefit of talking about health with another person is that through this conversation we may be directed to new possibilities such that our lives are changed. The psychotherapist does this as a matter of course (discourse). The medical doctor is expected to do this, but often ignores the symbolic meaning, and we have specific healing groups that refer to themselves as spiritual or religious. Yet, other than these formal healing encounters, we have the healing encounters of friendship (intercourse).

Each social contact has within it the potential for achieving change. Each offers alternative understandings and models alternatives for recovery within that relationship. Where we have difficulties is shown by Eva. She was talking from her understanding of her problem, with a set of understandings about the possibility of recovery that were incongruent with both general medical practice and psychological distress management. This is not to blame any party, simply to point out that with plurality we also have potentials for confusion. Expectations need to be congruent with the contexts within which they are expressed.

Same activity, different meaning

When I was a small boy my grandfather took me to the local park where he sat with his cronies and I played various games. To give himself some respite from me, he suggested that I ran around the bowling green. He would either time me to see how fast I could run or he would count how many circuits I completed. This was play for me and I would imagine myself to be some athletic hero of the day like Chris Brasher or Emil Zatopek.

Such play became sport as I grew up and started cross-country running. In my twenties I played other sports and ran, not only for the simple fun of it, but also because I wanted to improve my fitness; fitness to play sport that is, not as a health activity. In the culture of the East Midlands of England, health-care for men was something you did after your first heart attack and that included either smoking less or drinking less.

In my thirties I started to study again and as an aid to preparing for my examinations I began to run every day after studying. I enjoyed both the running and the studying. However, in my forties my father had his first heart attack and I began running again, not this time for enjoyment but as a hedge against angina. I soon stopped. The pleasure had gone from such activity. I was picking up more minor injuries 'jogging' than going for my daily walk. It did not help my father either.

Feeling good

If we take the same activity, in this case running, we can infer differing attributes to it and the benefits that it may have brought for my health. Biddle (1995) refers to this as the 'feel good factor'. Indeed, people had seen me running in my thirties and thought I was doing it for my health. This was quite false. I did it for the sheer pleasure of running like a boy and as a practical activity that would enable me to enjoy playing. It enabled a 'fit' identity, but this was an identity as a sportsman in a culture where being active in sport was part of an acceptable male identity. Only later did the same activity gain overtones of a health-care activity. It is precisely this aspect of understanding such an activity in relationship to a broader field of understandings and activities that is important when we consider health-care. The same activity is not always what it appears to be on the outside, there are rules of constitution.

The moral menu

As a final example I would like to refer again to the element of pleasure and how it is ignored in health-care thinking. A current debate has been about the implication of cholesterol in coronary heart disease (Evans *et al.* 1994) where eating a fatty diet is seen to be an unhealthy behaviour. A favourable way of eating has been proposed as the 'Mediterranean diet' that includes less fats, less meat, more fruit and vegetables and carbohydrate like breads and pastas. Again, in the spirit of academic benevolence, I have eaten in the Mediterranean and holidayed on a Greek island. Apart from the incidence of cigarette smoking that accompanied such meals and the intake of various fermented beverages, there were several cultural factors rarely mentioned in health-care directives about diet that might play a significant role.

First, the meals were slow affairs, often partaken within a large family group late in the evening. Second, the food was enjoyed as an activity among a series of activities that might include dancing or going for a stroll outside to take the evening air. Cultural setting and the temporality of eating seem to be forgotten in health-care descriptions of diet. The palpable enjoyment of the food, as an eating activity and as a social occasion, had little to do with a seemingly narrow concept of nutrition. Perhaps the reason for the failing inducements to change dietary habits (Meillier, Lund and Kok 1996; Nguyen, Otis and Potvin 1996) are simply that such inducements demonstrate a poverty of understanding in the nutritional argument concerning the human activity of eating together as a pleasurable activity. Eating is also a sensual activity. Hamilton *et al.* (1995) refer to vegetarians as eating from a moral menu and it is such a virtuous aspect of acceptable conduct that appears to pervade health-care arguments.

But pleasure is not enough. We have to locate this pleasurable activity within a meaningful social context. This has consequences that are personal and cultural, to which I refer as ecological (Aldridge 1998). Health is a constellation of activities as a complex praxis aesthetic.

Health as praxis aesthetic

Health-care arguments as presented by conventional medicine and many complementary medical initiatives are founded upon a charismatic ideology; that is, health is pursued for health's sake. The same goes for religion, life for a divine being's sake, or art, art for art's sake. However, health is predicated on the reality of the body. Health, religion and art are presented as metaphysical activities – they are above the physical realm. But like the body of work in terms of art products, the individual body in terms of physical health is subject to temporality and is not above the substantial plane of existence. Health is temporal and locally corporeal. There is a functional aesthetic relating to the performed body by which we recognize the outcome of healing. To be accepted as a performance, a *habitus* (Bourdieu 1993), there must be an audience and that returns us to the social field of the other and culture. It too is moral.

While body size and shape are aspects of personal identity, it is how the body is interpreted, the aesthetics of health beliefs that play an important role in forming identity. Such beliefs play an active part in how we recognize illness and what therapy form we choose (Aldridge 1992). Meanings provides a bridge between cultural and physiological phenomena. The diagnosis of a medical complaint is also a statement about personal identity (van der Geest 1994) and the stigma that may be attached to such an identity (Crossley 1995). Symbolic meanings are the loci of power whereby illness is explained and controlled. Such loci are now shifting from the educated health professionals to the increasingly better educated and health-conscious consumers.

Indeed, in the postmodern era there are ever-increasing producers of symbolic goods related to health. Various agencies, including consumer groups, now make claims for a healing legitimacy in competition with the orthodoxies of conventional medicine (although it appears sometimes that complementary medical agencies have been incorporated within the body of conventionality). The notion of alternative medicine, consumer groups, healing groups and self-care groups have struggled to liberate health from the grip of academic control and the monolith of conventional medicine. This has been linked to the development of individual autonomy whereby the health of the individual can be performed as he or she sees fit. Health has the potential of a style and form liberated from a subordination to conventional political and medical interests:

> The mass production of works produced by quasi-industrial methods – coincided with the extension of the public, resulting from the expansion of primary education, which turned new classes (including women) into consumers of culture. The development of the system of cultural production is accompanied by a process of differentiation generated by the diversity of the publics at which the different categories of producers aim their products. (Bourdieu 1993, p.113)

If we substitute 'health' for 'culture' and 'health-care' for 'cultural' in the previous passage, then we have an accurate description of the health-care market.

Definition of health in a cultural context

In our modern cultures several belief systems operate in parallel and can co-exist. Patients have begun to demand that their understandings about health play a role in their care and practitioners too are seeking complementary understandings. Health itself is a state subject to social and individual definition. What counts as healthy is dependent upon cultural norms. Health and disease are not fixed entities but concepts used to characterize a process of adaptation to meet the changing demands of life and the changing *meanings* given to living. Negotiating what counts as healthy is a process in which we are all involved, as are the forms of treatment, welfare and care which we choose to accept as adequate or satisfactory.

People do not merely accept the identities passed down by authorities. Instead, they construct their identities from various sources. Modern identity is eclectic. As in the age of Romanticism, when revolution demanded a new way of being, the primacy of the perceiver is once more being emphasized. Subjectivity becomes paramount, on the one hand reifying the individual, but on the other running the risk that the individual will become isolated. Indeed, while post-modernism is perhaps characterized by a revolt against authority and tends towards self-referentiality, its very eclecticism, which leaves the individual valued but exhausted of significance – what Gergen (1991) refers to as 'the saturated self'. Brewster-Smith (1994) suggests that the inflated potential for selfhood dislocated from traditional value sources increases the potential for despair. While individuals may rise to the challenge of pluralism, there are some who will seek to join groups that offer a form of reassurance in a given orthodoxy of beliefs and actions. The danger in modern Europe is that the romantic notion of indivi-dualism, becomes perverted into nationalism. The dislocated individual, seeking to construct his or her own identity, joins a group intent on the limitation of others' freedom of self-definition whereby he or she can maintain their own security. Consensus is fragile in a context where individual demands are reified.

Health as functional aesthetic

The notion of lifestyle appears to be important in describing modern approaches to health-care use and its delivery. In a Foucauldian sense, the self is not an assemblage of functional components, but a unified style of behaviour (Dreyfus 1987). However, this unified ideal is being challenged. Rather than there being a human nature, the postmodern, self-interpreting practice of being human enables varying natures. Identities are constructed and maintained each day, thus a performed identity and a functional aesthetic. In this sense the activity of healing is concerned not with restricting us to a one-dimensional sense of being according to an accepted orthodox world view, but the possibility for the interpretation of the self as new, albeit embedded as an identity within a particular culture. This is the idea of personality as *persona*, identity as mask that can be presented according to the situation. What we lose is the connection between what we are and what we present. It could well be that we are so busy presenting identities that we are failing to achieve any development of an inner content.

Therefore, we have expression of continuing dissatisfaction and feelings of emptiness; all site and no substance.

Individuals seek to make claims about their personal identity to someone else to whom they matter, that is, in interaction. Claiming to be a healthy, fulfilled, empowered, artistic or spiritual person is a way of presenting self that will elicit a response from others. Schwalbe (1993) interprets this action of deciding which identity to present and in how we present ourselves as one of moral agency. In modern descriptions of alternative healing, it is the body that is the stage for the interaction of the self and its interaction with culture. Thus the body becomes the moral arena and the moral performance itself. This sets the stage not only for displays of extravagant achievement but also for displays of distress. In anorexia nervosa, the body is the stage of a tragic drama that is personal, relational, moral and political.

Health as a performed art

If the big narratives of modernism are now being replaced by our own personal sets of meaning made locally with those with whom we live (Warde 1994), then we need to understand more about the person who sits before us in our consulting room. How that person creates an identity will be indicative of how that person will resolve his or her problems. How that person seeks to be identified will guide his or her health-care activities. Some will seek medications; others will imbibe herbal preparations; others will seek to be physically manipulated; others will seek to be psychically manipulated; yet others will exchange energies, both subtle and cosmic; some will search for the laying on of hands in a ritual way – whether from a medical doctor or a spiritual healer (both require their own brands of faith); some will sing to relieve their souls and others will jog for the heart's content. Each of these, the bodybuilder and the disciple, the artist and the atheist, the athlete and the allopath, will demand a recognition for whom they are as a person and for that recognition to be included in treatment decisions. Indeed, the route to treatment will be guided by an itinerary pertinent to personal identity. Health is something that is done, a performed art.

What we singularly fail to see is that our current thinking about health is dominated by a medical thinking that ignores much of the reality of the persons we intend to treat and support. Few people, when they are sick, respond by seeking a health-care practitioner (Andersen 1995). Perhaps even fewer consult a health-care practitioner about staying healthy. What we appear to do, outside of an academic life thinking about health-care and its discourses, is eat, drink, amuse ourselves, love our nearest and dearest, walk the dog, chase pieces of leather across fields (both dogs and football players), without thinking of medical consequences. Maybe our health-care assumptions are so narrow that they have little relevance for others who do not bow down at the altars of epidemiology and empiricism. Many lay appraisals of health-care activity seem be based upon holistic considerations that include feelings of mood and vitality (Andersen 1995). If changes of mood are ignored, or assessed as potentially pathological by health-care practitioners, and the philosophy of vitality is generally regarded as invalid in modern scientific medicine, then we should not wonder that few people come to us for help. If, as in traditional Chinese medicine, for example, health seeking becomes a pleasure, that sequesters 'a body that cannot only taste sweetness but be sweet, not only report painful symptoms, but also dwell on and cultivate the quiet comforts of health' (Farquhar 1994, p.493), then maybe we can understand that the seeking of a positive identity in a postmodern world is an activity which can be enjoyed without experts and the grand narratives of science and medicine. We may indeed have to learn to seek out those personal and local truths that our patients are themselves choosing to embody. This embodiment will be located in a culture that gains its meaning from the way in which pleasure is sought and distress is transformed. The field of health influences as they are played out in the community manifest themselves in the pleasured bodies of individual persons. The activities of those in turn influence the manifestation of the pleasurable culture in which they are embodied.

Lifestyle as commodity

Since the last decade of the twentieth century there has been a change in relationship between self and society. The individual is becoming dislocated from a traditional commitment to society, a disenchantment with the collective. A new type of commitment is being seen (Warde 1994). In a liberal ideology, individuals with enough disposable income are becoming personally responsible for their own identity and this is linked to lifestyle as commodity. Individuals are socialized in a postmodern society as consumers with a choice of lifestyles. While on the one hand our autonomy is restricted in the field of employment (if we can find employment), how we choose to define ourselves and with whom we choose to define ourselves is a matter of personal freedom. An anomaly of this situation is that personal perceptions of health, their own well-being and life satisfaction may be at odds with a health professionals' assessment of that individual's health status (Albrecht 1994).

The danger of this individual health lifestyle approach, when it assumes that health is the opposing pole of a health–illness construct, is that individuals are held as responsible for the causation of their own diseases (Kirkwood and Brown 1995) and lifestyle factors can be seen as the precursors, risk factors, of future illness (Armstrong 1995). Health becomes expressed as a moral debate concerning responsible citizens free from the intervention of doctors. This in turn masks the agenda of restricting access to limited resources. Rather than the sick being labelled as deviant, the sick become labelled as illegitimate users of provision. In England such a situation has occurred whereby advertisements in national newspapers have been taken out on behalf of a medical association requesting patients only to contact their doctor in an emergency. To whom does the individual turn for healing? It would be perverse to restrict access to conventional medical attention and at the same time refuse to legitimize the healing activities of other groups. Religious and spiritual healing have traditionally formed this cultural network of healing for the poor who have limited access to medical care.

Promoting and maintaining our health is one such choice in the plethora of consumer activities intimately related to our identity. The bodybuilder, eating efficiently for the production of a body mass, will consume differently from the computer freak who surfs the Internet and eats fast food for a fast lifestyle. Both will differ from the jogging yoghurt eater who consumes vegetables to purify his material self, reduce his cholesterol levels and meditates for the salvation of the planet. The young boy who was running for fun in my earlier example grew up to be the young man running for pleasure, who became the middle-aged man running for his life, who has become the old man sitting down and remembering what it was like. While the same activity prevailed through each episode, the needs being gratified are different (Montelpare and Kanters 1994; Tinsley and Eldredge 1995).

The implication of Bourdieu's work (see Randal Johnson's Preface in Bourdieu 1993) is that any analysis that overlooks the social grounds of aesthetic taste tends to establish a universal aesthetic and cultural practices that are in fact products of privilege; so it is of a privileged universal approach to health practice. A pure scientific understanding of medicine keeps necessity at arm's length. Daily life will always subvert such an health aesthetic: thus my call for a praxis aesthetic of health based upon the performed body located in social relationship and belonging to a culture of shared understandings. The sharing of understandings and the maintenance of relationship are also performed activities.

Implications for health promotion

I would like to consider three practical areas of health-care that relate to the previous arguments. All are subject to the charismatic ideology that assumes a monolithic perspective on health as applied by experts who know that is often based upon an hidden moral agenda.

The first concerns AIDS educational campaigns that are aimed at encouraging safe sex among gay men. Such educational material has assumed that there is an homogeneous culture to which gay men belong and that behavioural change will follow as a logical consequence from reasoned exhortation. Gold (1995) argues otherwise. There is not a safe sex culture in existence, and the encouragement to have safe sex has missed out on the reality of pleasure involved in sexual contact.

As mentioned previously, health-care rationale, for the individual, is not necessarily linked to a carefully planned strategy as health-care professionals like to believe. There are disparities between what people say they believe and what they do.

For some gay men, the constellation of sexual gratification, recreational pleasure and the maintenance of a particular lifestyle, tied up as it is with a gay identity, does not have health-care as a principal strategy for living, even in a climate of AIDS prevention. Human beings live, with optimism and zest, to enjoy life, not necessarily to prevent illness. Any interventions aimed at changing behaviour in gay men to promote a safer sex culture will need to accept that there are groups of men with differing lifestyles and expectations, some of whom may not be benign and benevolent towards a wider community.

Dieting

A second example is in the field of dieting and exercise as they are related to body shape. Females in Western industrialized cultures are not only expressing concern about their bodily shapes but are actively engaged in altering how they appear. The body is the interface between the woman herself, as a person, and her social identity. Feelings about the self are related to feelings about the body. They are not solely located in the body, but are concerned with how that body appears to others. A vast amount of time and money is spent on consumer activities related to this body image in terms of exercise activities, fashion and diet. Slimness has become popularly associated with elegance, self-control, social attractiveness and youth (Furnham, Titman and Sleeman 1994). Such descriptions are also the motivating factors associated with the sales pitch of many consumer products. While such personal lifestyles of dieting for fitness and the presentation of a powerful potent body may be health enabling, there is also the paradox that these very activities are involved in the generation of eating disorders. The encouragement of the excessive individualism, while promoting autonomy, may be at the expense of her integrity as a whole person. She is connected to a set of cultural values that threaten to destroy her health when disembedded from the relations that may offer a social meaning to her personal identity. This excessive emphasis on the individual body dislocated from the social body is classically reflected in the egoism explanation in Durkheim's explanation of suicide (Warde 1994).

Smoking

A third example is concerned with cigarette smoking in the young. While there has been a considerable impact on behalf of educational campaigns to curb adult smoking, those campaigns have failed to make any impact on the prevalence of young smokers (Lynch 1995). Lynch argues that this failure is because educational campaigns singularly fail to understand the reasons why young people smoke. These reasons may not be homogeneous and certainly will not follow the causal sensible logic of most health-care professionals. Image is seen as a powerful factor in influencing smoking behaviour, as is the need to be 'an individual'. Thus campaigns aimed to curb enjoyment, emphasizing a sensible conformity to an artificially constructed target group of adolescent smokers falsely assumed to be homogeneous, will be doomed to failure.

Individual understanding: Tailor-made health-care

We see that hedonism, the enjoyment of the body, the maintenance of a self-image and pursuing an active, seemingly healthy lifestyle can be both health promoting but in some circumstances deleterious to health. The pursuit of excessive individualism may lead to a disentanglement from social relationships that are vital to bringing some checks and balances to counter extremes of living that may prove to be deleterious. There is no easy reconciliation of this problem but we will see in the next chapter the way in which spirituality is an important factor in the treatment of alcoholism.

Our health-care endeavours must target small groups and individuals. There are no easy global solutions that can be applied from the top down. Struggling to understand the individual and those with whom he or she is bound is vital. If this is central to the practice of health-care in the consulting room, then it can surely be extended to our health-care reasoning.

The ramification of all this for health-care is that, instead of a top-down approach to its promotion, we must consider targeting interventions aimed at small groups in which individuals are embedded; this has been the underlying principle of church-based healing communities.

Lives that are performed

We have to understand how people 'do' their lives, not simply what they think and say about their lives. It is in the body that individual identity is expressed, and the body is the interface between the individual and society. It is what people do together that binds them to the groups with whom they perform their lives. This performance will involve lifestyle, leisure activities, exercise, dieting and dress. In this sense 'lifestyle' is not something that can be read about in books, it is an activity. Making sense of the world is an activity achieved through the body. Swimming cannot be learned about by reading about it, by gathering together a band of expert swimmers to tell you about their experiences, or by attending a conference of hydro-physicists. At some time we have to jump into the water and through experience do it. The body grasps what it needs to do. Having a teacher in the water certainly helps; so too with health and a change in 'lifestyle'. If we wish to encourage people to do something differently, we have to understand that it will be intimately connected with their identity as a person and those with whom that identity is validated. Health-care professionals are no longer the group with whom our patients wish to identify. With their rates of suicide, marital disruption and drug abuse who can blame them? Change is brought about by influencing small groups and understanding their way of being in the world. Religious and spiritual healing has indeed taken this approach. Through specific activities, private or public, means of healing are offered in which individuals can take part. Thus the body is performed, but in performative contexts; performative contexts that offer appropriate forms for bodily expressions.

Relationship is central for expression. Once relationship is lost, then the expressive quality of the performance is denied, and without relationship we lose the parameters for restraint. We saw this in women on a psychiatric hospital ward who mutilated themselves (Aldridge 1998). Once removed from meaningful social contexts, then mutilation increased. The expressive body is used to maintain relationship and extremes of expression may be amplified to regain relationship. How an individual realizes a personal identity, validated within a relationship, will be seen in the next chapter as central for the treatment of alcoholism.

Health beliefs and healing identities

With the postmodern challenge to orthodoxies, there appears to be a concurrent search for meaning in the face of chaos, loss, hopelessness and suffering. New efforts for lay involvement in medicine and the church and a call for spiritual (or wholistic) understandings of illness are the expressions of individual calls for such meaning according to individual belief. However, such descriptions are often careful to distinguish the belief in a transcendental reality, or a search for purpose and meaning, from a particular religious viewpoint. Where the grand narratives have disappeared, there seems to be an emergence of locally structured interest groups to meet the needs of individuals searching for shared meanings.

It is at the level of health beliefs where perhaps the most conventional forms of healing explanations take place. For black American women with AIDS (Flaskerud and Rush 1989), the sources of their illness and their remedies were classified as natural and supernatural. Prevention, prayer and spirituality were included in a treatment programme which incorporated traditional beliefs. This incorporation of modern and traditional has also been described in treating various ethnic groups throughout the world (Conway 1985; Dillon 1988; Griffith 1983; Loudou and Frankenberg 1976). What is important to learn from these experiences is that patients have concerns for the origins and meanings of symptoms that are important to them and for the way in which they may be healed.

Symbolic meaning plays an active part in disease formation, classification, the cognitive management of illness and in therapy (Kleinman 1973, 1978, 1980; Kleinman and Sung 1979; Lewis-Fernandez and Kleinman 1994). Such meanings provide a bridge between cultural and physiological phenomena. The diagnosis of a medical complaint is also a statement about personal identity (van der Geest 1994). Symbolic meanings are the loci of power whereby illness is explained and controlled. These symbolic meanings are often contained within particular ritual practices, hence the prohibition of spiritual healers in England from wearing white coats in hospitals. If such healers did wear white coats there would be a confusion of symbolic realities and hierarchies belonging to particular rituals of orthodox medicine. Griffith (1983) describes this cultural discrepancy in a church-based healing clinic which mixed both orthodox modern medicine and spiritual healing. Not only were there differences in healing realities, there were differences in rituals and in hierarchies of practitioners. While separate rituals may exist in parallel, it is another gigantic step to ask that they work in unison. Some authors see such unity as diluting the richness of the culture in that marginal practices will be medicalized and lose some of their vitality (Glik 1988).

It is a change in the sense of meaning of life which appears to characterize many reports of healing rituals. Marginalized individuals, the sick, the poor, the lonely and the elderly, are brought into a group context. For some participants this offers a way of self-expression and fulfilment within a social context, thereby ritually affirming the social worth of the individual (Griffith and Mahy 1984; Griffith, Mahy and Young 1986). Thus, some church-based healing groups are more concerned with lifestyle approaches rather than physical pathologies. From this perspective, sickness, when placed in the hands of a divine authority, releases the patients to a new form of living and integration within a community. For both individuals and groups, lifestyle choices have become an important factor in maintaining identity. However, rather than calling upon a divinity as ministered through the clergy or priesthood, such a divine agency is considered to be that of the self.

From various community groups, even within a single 'church', there is a growing demand for involvement in health issues and for initiatives in promoting a healthy lifestyle. Within the churches at large there are demands by the laity to be actively involved. What is being proposed is that individuals are allowed to minister to themselves with the support of informed advisers who can fulfil the role of facilitator. The idea of community health in these descriptions may be alluded to as an ecological context, but there is little reference to an immediate social or communal context.

However, the descriptions invoked to describe the process of healing and its effects are firmly located in cultural contexts. Concurrently, there is demand by individuals to construct their own identities (Spickard 1994), one of the elements of which may be a wish to be considered as 'spiritual'. Individual treatment regimes, 'growth' practices, techniques of self-realization are the exercise of individual choice whereby some like-minded individuals may form groups on an ad hoc basis. What counts as 'spiritual' is informed by culture as rules of constitution and how to be 'spiritual' is also informed by culture as rules of regulation (Aldridge 1998). Who legitimates such practices within a pluralist culture of health-care delivery is a continuing political discussion and indicative of liberalism in a democratic society (Aldridge 1990a).

The notion of lifestyle appears to be important in describing modern approaches to health-care use and its delivery. Healing is concerned not with restricting us to a one-dimensional sense of being according to an accepted orthodox world view, but the possibility for the interpretation of the self as new. In the next chapter I hope to demonstrate that this is the process of healing for the recovering alcoholic.

5

Lost and found
The perpetual story

The candle is not there to illuminate itself. (Idries Shah 1968)

This chapter is concerned with the body and how the pursuit of pleasure can become an activity that is far from pleasurable. Alcohol-related disorders are a major health-care problem in Western industrialized societies (Starrin *et al.* 1990), particularly when coupled with problems related to mental health in general and suicidal behaviour, in particular (Appleby 1992; Hawton *et al.* 1993; Henriksson *et al.* 1993). While we must not evade the social conditions under which alcoholism occurs (Brenner 1987; Elias 1996), it is the interface of the individual in relationship with the social that this chapter considers.

What kind of drinking is too much drinking? When we drink too much, albeit in the pursuit of pleasure, when does that drinking become a health-care concern? As soon as we start to describe any activity as being concerned with too much, then we assume that there are limits being set, that there are normative thresholds for what is adequate. The individual is judged and placed within a social and cultural context that says his or her behaviour is inappropriate. Consumption is regulated according to too much, as in alcoholism, or too little, as in anorexia nervosa. Reading the recommended medical literature on alcohol consumption, it is quickly apparent that the thresholds for consumption are constructed to maintain functional requirements at a social level of understanding and are concerned with control, thereby political and moral.

We saw in the previous chapter that pleasure, and bodily pleasure at that, is a feature of modern day health care. In a Foucauldian sense, where he writes about Greco-Roman contexts of pleasure in everyday life, bodily pleasure is a natural and proper activity (Foucault 1985). Going beyond 'natural limits', such that health is damaged, shows poor judgement or a lack of control (Smith 1999). Control, as we will see later, is to be a principle element in understanding the alcoholic, as in the latter stages of drinking control fails. Poor judgement is the basis of what was called 'sin'; sin simply being a matter of making poor judgements, of missing the mark. The metaphor commonly used is that of an archer missing the target as his mark; the target, in a religious sense, being an awareness of god. Thus losing or forgetting the long-term target of life, the achievement of god, is considered a sin. Particularly in the context of hedonism, where enjoyment is paramount, then our lives have another focus: the immediate without concern for the long term. Little wonder that talk of sin seems to be such a 'killjoy' attitude with high moral overtones. If, however, lack of control is the result of a disease, then it can no longer be thought of as a sin. It is no longer under personal influence. The sinner has become a sick person.

Failing to realize that daily life is to be directed towards a higher power means a loss of the transcendental context. The greater purpose of life is lost, albeit temporarily. In this sense a religious perspective has emphasized that we are all sinners constantly missing the point. Through spiritual awareness we are offered the hope of finding the way back and regaining that context. Unfortunately this understanding has become overloaded with such a moral overtone of condemnation by religious practices such that the point is indeed missed. When I mention sin in this chapter, I am not talking of a 'Deuteronomic formula of cause and effect: God rewards the righteous with blessings and punishes the sinful with suffering' (Parker 1997), but simply a loss of context, missing the point, falling out of the divine relationship; a metaphor for losing a particular consciousness. Some ancient traditions refer to this as being asleep (Khan 1974, 1983). It is part of the human state and something we all do.

The process of healing will entail the recovery of this consciousness. It is called a way of return in some spiritual systems. We are upon a path that returns us to consciousness, an awareness of unity with the divine. The problem is that each religion attempts to ensure that there is only one way back and that it has the only way. In a postmodern world this is no longer acceptable. There are many ways to return, each according to the seeker. Unfortunately, while a postmodern approach accepts that there many paths to return, the authority of a teacher who would enable this return as expert is denied.

Not condemnation

As we shall see later, the change of moral attitude towards drinking as sin to alcoholism as a disease is central to the treatment of alcoholism by Alcoholics Anonymous. We will also read that by reminding the drinker of a divine power, life is given another meaning and purpose and she can be freed from her addiction. This is described in the literature as a spiritual approach and contains the necessary elements of transcendence and meaning that we saw in Chapter 2.

The original meaning of sin, as we have seen, was a simple reminder of a purpose in life. It was not meant as a condemnation, simply a reminder for orientation, like the athlete who breaks her training for an extra meal when her long-term aim is to win an Olympic medal. Unfortunately the Church made it a matter of moral condemnation separating the bad from the good; the bad were the sinners and the good were inevitably male and part of the priesthood. This situation of taking the moral high ground is repeated in current secular contexts where high priestesses and priests of health exhort us to watch what we eat, drink and inhale. With a shift towards the body as the exhibition site for personal identity, as evidenced by perfect shimmering health, unpolluted, fat and alcohol free, we have a material concept of sin that any ascetic would be proud of, with perhaps the exception that the body as healthy object is itself being enjoyed. Such narcissism too would be a sin, losing focus on the divine by dwelling in the body. A central problem of the concept of sinner is that it needs a judge who is pure to set the standards of the others, therefore, the introduction of separation and a loss of unity.

Demonstrating lack of control can also be seen as not submitting to social control; then we have not a sick individual but a subversive person. The sin is ascribed to the sinner by society; he is either judging poorly according to social standards or rejecting those standards. The question remains of control for what purpose? What the sick, the sinner and the subversive have in common is their failure to comply with control. While we may try and locate that loss of control in the individual, and it certainly is so physically located in alcoholism, control is a systemic phenomenon (Bateson 1978). By locating the problem in the individual, we systematically delude ourselves of a social distress. A drinker becomes an alcoholic. He has a biography. Distress has escalated. While the alcoholic drowns his distress in alcohol, we also encapsulate the manifestation of distress in the drinker. This is not to deny that there are drinkers, simply to say before we assign culpability, that we understand our part in that process. As in individual suicidal behaviour, we have to see collectively how we have become the architects of despair.

'Although we are many, we are one body' would seem to be an adequate injunction for a social awareness that diverts blame from the individual as well as being a spiritual injunction collectively. In a postmodern context, however, we can interpret this as 'Although we are many, we are all parts of a temporary presentation' or 'Although we are many, we can all partake of alternative identities as networked *atavars*'. This is not a resolution of Cartesian dualism, simply a one-sided emphasis on mind as disembodied virtual reality. Body as body, the sensual filled experienced, that which eats drinks and fornicates, is located in presentation as a cultural ideal. Body as imperfect flesh, flat, flatulent and fallen, is denied. The drinker, the suicidal slasher, the self-starver, remind us that the body is indeed dying in postmodern society. Body is being starved of its vital spirit. Spirituality may be used as a term in a postmodern context but it fails to become incarnate. It remains the metaphysical illusion that postmodernism seeks to deny.

Both Bourdieu and Foucault regard the body as influencing social structure as well as being influenced by such structures. Bodily functions are regulated as part of a civilizing process and as this process proceeds the body becomes increasingly bounded, isolated and separated from other bodies. Self-control has become mapped onto the body as bodily control where will, power and energy are used to control the body and give shape to a life (Lawton 1998). Self-assertion and a fighting spirit become hallowed properties of the modern personality. These regulated bodies provide models for cultural ideas. But where do the weak in spirit, the poor, the disabled, the imperfect, the meek and the careworn fit into this perfected ideal?

A stigmatized identity

Poor health, resulting in a damaged body from loss of control, also has implications for a stigmatized identity. The personal becomes social. We see this in the process of becoming alcoholic where the bodily toll brought about by drinking and the ramifications for personal relationships bring about the ascription of the condition 'alcoholic'. In Nicosia's (1983) biography of Jack Kerouac, we read that it is Kerouac's increasing incontinence and his impotence that provide the clues to how serious the condition is other than his bouts of drinking. As in the elderly, losing bladder control is taken as a sign that the person is indeed in need of a specific medical care and has overstepped a boundary of personal presentation that brings his social status into question.

Achieving the status 'alcoholic' is a performative practice, the embodied person in a social context of distress. Changing this situation, relieving distress, is dependent upon a change from a negative to a positive identity. Bringing about this change is achieved through the social and the personal. However, before we embark upon the process of healing, I need to continue my story of sin and poor judgement (although I enjoyed it at the time) from the previous chapter.

If the reader remembers, I was at the beer festival enjoying myself. At ten o'clock the beer halls close during the festival, so we all trooped off to a pub. The conference was at an end and the organizers were intent on enjoying themselves. Being personally invited by the organizers to attend the party, it would have been churlish to refuse to go along. It would also have broken the habits of a lifetime. Anyway, the night was still full of promise and it became harder to say 'no' and easier to say 'yes'. The reader will have identified either positively or negatively with this narrative by now. A moral identity is being performed and, as we will read, it only gets worse. But before things can get worse, they have to get better. The pub proved to be an exciting place where all sorts of exotic characters visited. The group I was with started to loosen up and we told each other stories about our lives and work; altogether the very stuff of social life in a 'wet' culture (Eisenbach-Stagl 1998). Things were so good that when the pub closed at one o'clock in the morning we decided to adjourn to the bar of the hotel where the majority of colleagues were staying.

An attraction of this bar was that it replicated a South Sea island with decorated huts and waitresses in grass skirts and coconut brassieres. The crowning glory was the cocktails, which at this time of the morning had become cheaper. It was happy hour! At three o'clock it was time for the party to break up. A taxi was called, the fare was paid and I was sent to my hotel. The taxidriver was told where to go by my hosts as by then my bilinguality was a fleeting faculty and even monolinguality was severely challenged. The performed body was considerably incapacitated and uncoordinated.

Upon arrival at the hotel I collected my keys and went to my room on the sixth floor. It may have been the seventh but I cannot remember. Anyway, on approaching my room at the end of the corridor, I was aware of another person coming towards me and that person was certainly the worse for wear regarding drink. The nearer I got to my room, the nearer he got to me. So, being a non-hero by conviction, I retraced my steps and telephoned hotel security. They promptly sent two guards, this being an international hotel keen to retain its sense of security. As we approached my room, I was relieved to see that the drunk was returning too, but he also had company. They were not deterred by my guards and seemed set on confrontation. At this point the security guards, far from being anxious, became amused. At the end of the corridor was a mirror and the undeterred drunk and his cronies approaching the door were me and my guards.

Good taste is fragile

For Merleau-Ponty (1962) the body is a setting in relation to the world. We are simply a 'world' that begins as body, it is the starting point of perception. But this body is also performed for others, with others, and is informed by other bodies. We have a sense of taste and 'good taste', as a social sense that we saw in the previous chapter. We have a sense of taste as the pleasure of drinking beer, as my story tells, and of propriety in not having too much to drink. What we include in such narratives, like my trip to the Munich beer festival and, more appropriately, what we leave out, is concerned with the maintenance of a moral identity that is social. This identity is fragile and has to be maintained. If I were to repeat that experience too often then I would be in danger of being seen not just as a 'social drinker' but as addicted. Repeat the experience often enough and I would be in serious danger of enjoying myself or very, very tired. According to the milieu where this story is recounted, either I am a social drinker to be invited along to the next party or an unreliable colleague whose employment is questionable. Where and when drinking becomes a problem depends upon the social ascription of obligations that remain unfulfilled. It is also a problem when what was once enjoyable becomes distressing and the ability to stop drinking itself fails. Pleasure can become harmful. When repeated pleasurable activities incrementally fail to satisfy, then perhaps we have the basis for addiction. As Benedikt (1996, p.575) writes, 'True addictions not only compel us to repeat the act of "consuming" them by delivering pain when we do not, but the amount of pleasure they provide each time wanes.'

As you the reader can imagine, to return to the story, I awoke the next day to the sound of jackhammers and heavy machinery in what must have been a major construction project taking in part in the next room. Not only that, someone was busy ringing all the bells of every cathedral in the northern hemisphere, and ringing them inside my head. It was of course the telephone clamouring with a wake-up call and the beginnings of a hangover. As I moved to answer the telephone, nothing happened. The sounds continued but no movement: Negative locomotion. Not even a twitch. Fortunately this was temporary, but in the milliseconds between the paralysis and the movement an awful lot can happen cognitively.

Van Manen (1998) writes about the need to find a liveable relationship with the body. We experience our bodies silently. It is, and we need no awareness of it; we and it are one. Yet when that fragile relationship is disturbed, we no longer forget the self as being embodied. We are no longer at ease; the subjectified body becomes identified as an object. Life is challenged by pain, as we shall see below. Stiffness, pain were foremost; the 'taken for grantedness' (van Manen 1998) of a healthy body was gone. My hangover, then, was a fall from grace. The body was no longer taken for granted. It was no longer silent.

Pain as restricted consciousness

The body is the location of a performed identity, both personal and social. It is the arena where both fulfil their roles. On its surface we clothe, decorate, paint and pierce as personal expression and social sign. We have the positive expression of a created reality with the potential for unifying internal and external. The body, when used, becomes a liberating vehicle for achieving and expressing new forms of consciousness. As both Merleau-Ponty and Bourdieu suggest (Burkitt 1998), thought is not simply structured by mind but is learned bodily actions and habits, a set of learned dispositions within a social context. Thus we have a performed sensory body that has a repertoire of actions. Health too can be seen as a repertoire of performed actions.

Distress as performed in the context of the other

Some of these bodily actions will be used to express and manage distress. These are learned and negotiated within a social context. The body is the expressive site of pain, the embodiment of disability and the incorporation of chronic sickness.

In this sense, pain is a restriction of consciousness. It prevents a transcendence of the performed body. We become aware of a body performance that is usually silent. We perform our bodies unaware of the body itself. Health may be seen as not being aware of the body and being free to achieve the perception of the other, the antithesis of postmodern health-care narcissism. We are released to relationship. Pain, and the anticipation of pain, are restrictions on relationship. Pain removes us from interaction with the other and prevents us from knowing the other through contact. This too is part of the reason for traditional injunctions against becoming too aware of the body. By concentrating on the material presence of ourselves, we forget the other, the other as human and the other as divine, and thereby lose our purpose. We become self-centred. Indeed in Western thought we have developed notions of individual determination and autonomy about the body and what we do with it. In a Biblical sense, however, the body does not belong to the individual but 'is given to man by God as a trust to respect and preserve' (Walters 1999).

This process also works in reverse. When pain prevents contact with others, then the other is preserved in his purity from the deviant, the unclean, the tainted. We keep the disabled and the sick segregated.

Meaningful gestures in the healing drama

Symptoms, from a performative perspective, can be seen as gestures of communication that perform the self for others. Symptoms call forth a response from others that will be elicited as care and formalized as treatment. These symptoms, as significant symbolic gestures, have to be codified by particular approaches to treatment and we call this 'medicine', 'unconventional medicine' or 'healing', according to the cultural context of health-care delivery. These are cultured expressions in a repertoire of healing presented as performances and interpreted socially. Performances engage other actors in the production of a healing drama. Any dramatical performance is dependent upon the repertoire of roles available and such roles are legitimated according to the context in which they are presented. The ascription of legitimacy to the performance of symptoms is a central process of becoming sick or, as we shall see, becoming labelled as deviant. The process is cultural and political. We can say the same regarding the process of recovery. At the interface is an aspect of the self that is fragile. If the postmodern self is indeed the presentation of a cultural ideal, then the discrepancy between the presented self, when suffering, and the ideal as perfect is perhaps the source of the current dilemma of mental health.

Pain as forgetting

Pain is determined within a context of meanings (Zborowski 1952; Zola 1966). If spirituality is the process by which meanings are sought and transcended then pain inhibits the achievement of transcendental meanings. That is, its very restriction is in that we fail to be exposed to new contacts which may allow us to change.

In palliative care, the treatment of pain, such that pain is forgotten, is central in allowing the patient to complete the process of dying. Achieving the stages of awareness necessary to die are inhibited by pain. Pain relief needs to be seen in the projected category of a patient's life. The use of medical substances to deny pain in other contexts actually prevents the transformations necessary for living. In addiction this denial becomes as handicap. Existential pain is palliated. Spiritual authors consider alcohol as a veil over the soul, restricting awareness. Palliation derives from the Latin *palliare*, to put a cloak or mantle over suffering. So it is with pain relief when it is necessary in context. Any one of us who has experienced post-operative pain will know how necessary relief is. But when that pain relief prevents transformation, when pain is denied its purpose, then we have addiction. Addiction prevents a person from developing. The necessary transcendence that can be achieved with others is handicapped. The addict becomes isolated, further veiling himself from the influences of change, whether these be externally social or the healing impulses within himself. This social aspect stimulating an internal spiritual response has been the central plank of Alcoholics Anonymous.

Pain is valuable. It expresses a message that all is not well. Identifying the source of that message, as performed in pain, is the important part of the treatment encounter. What is necessary to understand is the life context in which pain is located. Palliation, in the trajectory of the dying, achieves the setting for transformations that are recognized as spiritual. Conversely, palliation for the alcoholic, when it masks the source of suffering, prevents transformations that are vital. Removing pain through the abuse of alcohol or other chemicals, without an understanding of underlying distress, is a denial of the soul's need for transformation. It denies the trajectory that every life has by limiting consciousness. Indeed, addiction seems to be the attempt to fulfil a personal need inappropriately such that satisfaction is never achieved. As we have seen earlier, if the individual is identified as the material location of social distress, fulfilment is misplaced from its social locus. This is pain as forgetting, ignoring the source because the solution would be political in emphasizing the social grounds of distress.

Falling from grace

A religious realization of the spiritual imperative is to achieve a sense of a higher self. This has been at the heart of the Gnostic tradition (Martinez III 1998). The Gnostic tradition emphasizes a direct relationship within the divine and the possibilities of immediate spiritual knowledge. The small secondary egotistical self of everyday life, the core of the 'Me Generation', is abandoned in favour of a higher self connected to a greater unity and a sense of selflessness. This is embodied in many religious teachings that talk about the death of self, not suicide, but a death of the *selfish*, sometimes referred to as the secondary *personality*. In some religious movements this is translated into the concept of being born again into a new life with a different spiritual awareness. From a Gnostic tradition, humanity is seen as the incarnation of a divine life and the study of humanity is a religious quest for understanding. Meanings are transcended through the search for an understanding of what it is to be human.

Anyone studying human beings whether she is a social scientist at a conference or by waking up each morning, getting the children off to school and cycling to work, recognizes that not only do we, as human beings, have an unlimited capacity for creativity and an ability to take care of ourselves, but a corresponding capacity for self-destruction, and a self-destruction that involves others. We literally fall out with those with whom we live and love. This falling out is a falling out of relationship; the old concept of a loss of grace. It is the basis of isolation. We become uncoupled not only from the social, the embodied other, but from the contexts in which we can perform and negotiate an identity that is the self. In this way we become uncoupled from the potentials that are our selves. Our options are reduced and the sense of self is restricted. The reparation of this situation is the opposite, literally 'falling in'.

Refugees within the soul

Spiritual traditions have also maintained that there is a connection to a higher or true self, sometimes known as a knowledge of the heart; not a literal organic heart, but a part of us which is at the core of being human and lends us identity. We realize that we are alienated from this higher self and become not only isolated socially without ourselves but individually within ourselves; literally refugees within our own souls. While the body may be the ground for worldly existence, the self that transcends that existence is veiled and then we perform identities which are damaging; damaging because we are cut off from those relationships that offer transcendence. It is this situation that we find in alcoholism. The drinker not only cuts himself off from social relationships that are potentially helpful, he also maintains an identity that systematically damages those relationships that remain. Furthermore, it is not only a social ecology that is disturbed. Within himself, he cuts himself off from any personal means of change. Bringing about change in this situation of hopelessness has been at the centre of Alcoholics Anonymous and is based on acknowledging that contact with a higher self is necessary and this is achieved through relationship, transcending the smaller self to a new identity.

Deviance, disease and the status sick

A social expectation of the sick person is that if he wishes to retain the status sick then he needs also to hold the restoration of health as a primary role (Parsons 1951). The drinker seemingly fails to fulfil this by virtue of what he is. He cannot be regarded as 'sick' as he will not partake of healing. The bridges of the road to restoration are swept away by floods of alcohol and the storms and vagaries of life. If he is not sick, then he is deviant, and thereby we have a moral condemnation of the drinker.

The ascription of illness is based upon norms of behaviour. These norms are negotiated, and this negotiation is established from a repertoire of possibilities, as we read earlier. While these possibilities are social, they are also individually embodied. This process becomes organic in the ecology of the person in his environment of significant others. As individuals we negotiate within ourselves tolerances for healthy functioning such that we remain intact as human beings. Yet these tolerances are not simply contained within ourselves, we live our lives with others. The tolerances of functioning for the maintenance of health are also negotiated socially. Therefore, it is possible to maintain a social context, yet engage in acts that are self-damaging. We see this in self-mutilation and attempted suicide where acts of mutilation and poisoning, as short-term strategies, serve a positive function within families and psychiatric hospital wards (Aldridge 1998). We have the same process in anorexia nervosa (Malson 1999). Adaptation to a social requirement may be damaging to the individual if he adapts his tolerances to include the performance of damaging behaviours to ameliorate distress. As Bateson (Bateson 1972) writes:

> It will be noted that the possible existence of such a positive feedback loop, which will cause runaway in the direction of increasing discomfort up to some threshold (which might be on the other side of death), is not included in conventional theories of learning. But a tendency to verify the unpleasant by seeking repeated experience of it is a common human trait. It is perhaps what Freud called 'the death instinct'. (Bateson 1972, p.299)

As Canguilhem suggests (Greco 1998a), health is distinguished from illness by the range of circumstances which an organism can afford to function normally. The state of illness is not a deviation from healthy norms but is a regulation of the organism by a restricted range of tolerance. As we shall see later, although the tolerance for alcohol increases in the course of alcoholism and physiological thresholds of adaptation are indeed widened, at times beyond physiological integrity, within a repertoire of distress management, possibilities are severely reduced to one option, drinking.

By adapting to external norms, the individual loses his personal agency and this results in a state of dis-ease. Indeed by restricting internal tolerance to external demands and losing a necessary balance by ignoring or subverting those internal demands, we have the process of pathology: literally, *pathos* as the way of pain and suffering. It is also a loss of meaning and purpose. From what we have read until now concerning the process of being healthy, it is also a loss of performance. This process may be adapting to a virus, to a pollutant, to a relationship or to a tyrant. In attributing the status sick or deviant to a person, then we have to consider the performative context of the health care system in which symptoms are presented and the possibilities that are offered for treatment. From this perspective, alcoholism has been increasingly seen as a disease.

Alcoholism as a constructed disease

A medical approach would have us believe that it considers alcoholism as morally neutral. Alcoholics are the way they are, not because of failures in social control but because of predispositions that are genetic or environmentally caused. May (1997) locates the label of 'alcoholic' being constructed as a disease in the mid-nineteenth century. Habitual drunkenness was no longer a matter of moral volition but biologically determined. Previously the great epidemics of the eighteenth century were attributed to the uncontrolled appetites of the labouring masses. A shift occurs in the attribution of the problem from the labouring masses to a personal identity reconstructed through medicalization (p.172). Drunkenness became the product of specific pathologies, not, like my night out in Munich, as the result of appetite or indulgence. Thus, the individual becomes absolved of guilt and has the opportunity to be recognized as 'sick' (May 1997; Rothschild 1998). Cunningham, Sobell and Sobell (1996) locate this change in the 1960s when there was an attempt to change public attitudes to alcohol from blame and punishment to concern for treatment.

Although alcoholism has become medicalized as a disease, we still have a moralizing stance regarding health. Mehta and Farina (1997) remind us that, in the case of mental health, the disease label 'sick' does not mitigate the stigma. Indeed, from a postmodern all-jogging, aerobic, fitness studio, 'you are what you eat', non-alcohol, cigarette-free, holistic perspective, becoming 'sick' is evidence of an immoral life and a poor scrutiny of the body. Becoming sick is to adopt a damaged identity expressing an irresponsible lifestyle. Morality returns with a vengeance in the New Age. There is sickness and 'sickness'.

Disease as metaphor

The concept of disease was vital in the development of Alcoholics Anonymous (Kurtz 1979). Steffen (1993) discusses the notion of disease as metaphor emphasizing the concept of disease as a cultural construct. Disease was used within Alcoholics Anonymous 'in a metaphorical sense as a strategy for action (p.29)' that has now, in medical terms, gained a material reality.

Alcoholics Anonymous introduced the concept of alcoholism as an allergy of the body and therefore *like* a disease. But this notion of a bodily allergy was also linked to that of a mental obsession (Kurtz 1979). It is the concept of a mental obsession which implies a far greater potential for action 'that permits a characterisation of alcoholism primarily as a spiritual disease which must consequently be treated with a programme for spiritual awakening (p.130)'. By emphasizing both elements of this metaphorical perspective we are released from the concept of medical disease to disease as metaphor, that is, *like a* disease. This will have implications for treatment.

The benefit of the 'alcoholism is sin' metaphor is that it allows people eventually to be freed. In the evangelical roots of the Alcoholics Anonymous movement, we see the principle of sinners being set free from the bondage of drinking. The medical fallacy has been to take the metaphor of disease literally, failing to see that the metaphor of 'sin' applied to alcoholism is a way of presenting self in the world that allows flexibility of understanding and for the possibility of healing. In old-fashioned terminology, sin can be redeemed, the sinner can be saved. From a disease perspective, acutely sick people can be cured but the chronic sick cannot. It is in the nature of chronicity that it remains so, and alcoholism is deemed to be a chronic disease.

How we label the problem, as disease or deviance, is important for establishing healing possibilities. Ford (1996) emphasizes that for life changes to take place the sufferer has to see that these changes can take place. If I suffer from an incurable disease, 'alcoholism', then I become powerless in the face of my addiction. Faced with a genetic make-up that predisposes me to such a problem, then how can I bring about a constitutional change? The alcoholic becomes not only a victim of his past but a victim of his own biology. If I am a sinner, like everyone else, then there is always the possibility that I can be saved. While I might be a victim of my own past biography, as we have seen an identity that is authored, my future biography may be authored somewhat differently, not as one of victim but as one set free.

We have to remember here that sinner is simply being used as a sense of relationship. The sinner has fallen out of a relationship with that which is cosmic. We could say that he has ignored his relationship within an ecosystemic pattern. This is not a causal relationship in that sin causes disease, simply that we suffer if we fall out of relationship. If we lose a friend or partner, it hurts. If we lose our relationship with the divine, cosmic, or whatever we wish to name it, then we suffer. In the Christian Bible there is the story of Jesus healing a blind man and his followers asked if it was because of the sins of the man or of his parents that he was blind. The reply was that it was neither. Blindness was not caused by sin. If so, then neither is alcoholism. But blindness, as suffering, did have in a Biblical sense a purpose through which a cosmic significance might be revealed. In this sense, as sinners we are not to be condemned but welcomed as a source of understanding, as a reminder of the need to return to a divine relationship. It is also a reason why there will never be a world without suffering. It is the human condition to suffer. Yet through suffering we are reminded of the responsibilities we have for each other and of the divine.

Not what it is, but what does it mean?

If a benefit of the concept of disease has divorced thinking about sickness from the metaphysics of evil (Greco 1998b), then we have to consider what heuristic value the concept of disease has. The danger is that instead of existing as a performed being, the individual become sedimented as a fact. He is an alcoholic. He achieves a stigmatized identity. In doing so the possibility of being interpreted in a new way is lost. As we saw earlier, the performance of a new identity is based on acting with others. Once those acts become facts then we are limited existentially. A repertoire of performance becomes limited, as does relationship. The meaning of living is sedimented into a restricted performance that precludes the possibility of transformation. By saying a person has a chronic disease we bury the idea that is necessary for his recovery; the idea that the condition should not be there (Greco 1998b).

Relationship as a lived reality

The advantage of the concept of a performed self is that performance must be interpreted anew in each context. Therapeutic activity will be one of those contexts of performance offering new interpretations, proposing the idea that the condition of being sick no longer serves a purpose, the purpose is being achieved. Meanings can be negotiated, transmitted and embodied. Thus we have the actuality of healing that offers the possibilities for transcendence by virtue of the presence of the other. It is this presence of the other, a fellow sufferer, that is also at the centre of Alcoholics Anonymous. It is a return to a new relationship, not as an abstract ideal but as a lived reality. It is also a move away from the notion that there is a world out there to be revealed and an insistence on a world that is being performed, with others.

I am not taking a radical constructivist position here in this book. There is a physical world out there. Minerals, plants and animals had their lives before human beings existed and from which we evolved. We are part of that natural world. However, there is a world of consciousness in which we partake as human beings that we construct. We perform and interpret our human condition. It is at this level I am writing here in terms of a performed reality. How that total realm of consciousness, in all its myriad manifestations, is realized and achieved as a *unity* is the goal of spiritual understanding.

The benefit of using the metaphor of a constantly improvised identity is that living becomes like jazz. Each one of us has a repertoire of themes by which we are recognized. We improvise these with others. Some themes may become standards, other themes fall away. Each performance exists for the moment and then fades. We are transient beings, existing and then dying in the moment. We are revived, performing ourselves anew in new situations with other players. Life no longer needs to be clutched at as an object. Life as a lived reality is improvised in the moment. The themes in the repertoire are the consolation that give us some consistency. That we share themes with others is what we may call culture. Therapy may be a reminder to us that there are common themes but it is an individualized repertoire that we create and perform. Sickness is when a form is retained that no longer serves our purpose as living creatively.

We also add created themes to the broader repertoire that we call culture. Locating distress in culture alone is a determinism that fails to ring true for the individual, just as locating the problem in the individual alone ignores her social being. How each influences the other, while complex, is vital to understand in the process of interpretation. I am not giving either priority, rather directing us to a constellation of understandings that can best be assessed in their pragmatics.

Malady

Perhaps it is possible to introduce the concept of malady here. As we have seen from Merleau-Ponty and Bourdieu, it is habitus that is paramount. The word malady is built upon the same Latin root, *habere*. It means to hold, to occupy or possess, and this can be nuanced in malady as being unwell or ill kept. Drinking may be harmful but is not necessarily sedimented as a disease. It can be seen as a habitus, a way of performing in the world, a malady. In the following section regarding deviance, it is the stage in a systemic process when the ascription of 'alcoholic' is made to one person that fixes the thresholds for the tolerance of distress within that person. The alcoholic 'holds' or possesses a restriction within himself. He literally incorporates distress. This process itself is as toxic, systemically, as the alcohol.

But holding can also mean that there can be a letting go. Malady is not a fixed identity like a sickness, it is a holding of a problem for identification in a location of distress. Unfortunately, in our systems of categorizing we mistake the location for source and this localization becomes fixed. In suicidal behaviour, one person necessarily becomes the articulator of systemic distress. Through her biography, she becomes *the* articulator of that systemic distress and herself progressively distressed when relief fails. Thus the holding function of the presentation of symptoms becomes fixed within her. She becomes sick. She embodies distress. My suggestion is that the same process happens in alcoholism and that the problem with naming it as a disease is that it fixes a location and loses the process.

This is not to deny that there is such a thing as disease with recognized pathogens that has a location in a corresponding organic or bodily milieu. However, we see in the renaissance of tuberculosis and polio that disease can be located in a causal framework which is both social and political irrespective of its expression in the individual.

The opposite is to encourage the process of healing and lose the stigma of the disease. This is complicated by the fact that becoming healthy is not so easily categorized, other than as a negative 'not sick', 'not drinking', 'dry'. Indeed, maybe the reason that we fail to categorize health is just that we do not wish to locate it, it is a moveable feast. Similarly, any attempt to determine health as a healthy sporty body in the contemporary Western idealized form (Lawton 1998) appears to be moralistic and itself damaging in its ramifications (Liebermann 1995; Malson 1999).

Alcoholism as deviance

The axis of responsibility for alcoholism is drawn as part of a social process of construing drinking behaviour in context. In Western industrialized cultures, the imputation of responsibility is made on the grounds of how the state of illness is achieved (see Figure 5.1). This can be seen in the way that some infections, as in venereal disease, are judged by the means of infection. In conditions such as obesity, due to overeating, or heart disease, due to careless exposure, then illness behaviour is held in a different light to those same states ascribed to socially legitimated causes, e.g. hormonal imbalance or genetic defect. Significantly for these states, the co-operation with treatment and the motivation to recover is considered important. It can be seen from the label 'drinker' that the person engaged in such behaviour is violating an important rule by being responsible for his own state. If alcoholism is the result of a genetic defect, a physiological propensity or even an allergy, it can be labelled as a disease and is morally neutral. But being labelled 'alcoholic' is a stigmatized identity, no matter how we view a disease status.

We see the same process in anorexia nervosa. If drinking is a moral condemnation of too much consumption, then anorexia is a condemnation of too little consumption. Both are poles of a social ascription to how consumption is to be controlled and how bodily control, the totem of postmodernism, is to be maintained. For both processes the axis of responsibility is located within a deviant person.

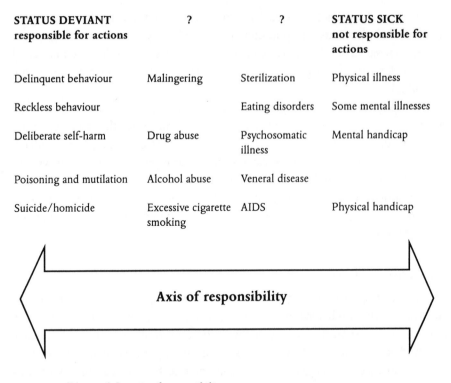

STATUS DEVIANT responsible for actions	?	?	STATUS SICK not responsible for actions
Delinquent behaviour	Malingering	Sterilization	Physical illness
Reckless behaviour		Eating disorders	Some mental illnesses
Deliberate self-harm	Drug abuse	Psychosomatic illness	Mental handicap
Poisoning and mutilation	Alcohol abuse	Veneral disease	
Suicide/homicide	Excessive cigarette smoking	AIDS	Physical handicap

Axis of responsibility

Figure 5.1 Illness and the axis of responsibility

Deviance as normality

Not all theorists regard deviance negatively, as catastrophic or pathological. Families require deviance to maintain homeostasis. Deviance becomes the creative stuff of evolution in social systems and if that deviance does not naturally arise a family will induce a member to break its rules. Once deviance appears, then a family will develop rules for sustaining it. Eating and drinking are natural. Over-eating, undereating and overdrinking are contained within family boundaries.

The usefulness of deviance was noted by Durkheim (1958) who pointed out that upright citizens develop functional feelings of cohesiveness when a criminal offender is caught and punished. In this way a common perspective and collective conscience is constituted. Erikson (1966) draws attention to the idea of a necessary deviance, that once one type of deviance is controlled then another type of deviance is likely to take its place. This view is reflected by Markush (1974) who describes a number of mental epidemics throughout the centuries which last for a period affecting many people and then disappear, only to appear in another form at a later date.

These authors stress that deviance is required in social systems because it serves several important positive functions. Deviant behaviour is induced, if not arising spontaneously, sustained and regulated within a social context. Erikson's (1966) theory suggests that the occurrence of deviant behaviour in a family is a natural part of the role differentiation process. Just as a family needs an emotional specialist or an organizer, so it requires a deviant. This suggests a construing of deviant–normal where family members can occupy such opposing poles for the necessary purpose of family change.

Defining values

The presence of deviant behaviour and accompanying sanctions serves an important purpose of defining normative boundaries. Deviant behaviour exemplifies the kinds of action that are not allowed and sanctions show what will happen if such acts occur. From a psychosomatic perspective, illness also has a purpose (Greco 1998a). It leads those involved to consider the values of life. These are varying reflections on the theological argument that the human condition is suffering and that suffering reminds us of the need to return to another unifying consciousness.

Individuals and families must negotiate their normative boundaries to promote predictable interaction. To do this, Erikson argues, families consistently apply sanctions to, not rejection of, a deviant member. Families seldom permanently stop deviant behaviour but maintain it at a level which promotes change and we see this in the literature relating to alcoholism (Cutter and Cutter 1987). The rate of change and escalation and severity of drinking are critical. It is this notion of applying sanction to but *not* rejecting the family member that is critical in considering self-damaging behaviours within their relational context (Aldridge 1998). Isolation is a significant factor in the process of becoming an alcoholic and rejection plays its part in such isolation. Drinking becomes an activity that is seen as 'deliberate self-harm'. Causal factors are attributed away from a social ecology to a location within the person. The drinker becomes an alcoholic.

Deviation is accepted when the deviation is limited in scope and when it does not pervade the whole person's being, when deviation is perceived as unstable and susceptible to change, and when deviance occurs in areas that are not central to a family's values. Alcoholism transgresses these rules. It pervades the whole person's being and threatens central values of life and death of cohesion and identity. When family members begin to see the phenomenon not as deviant behaviour but as evidence of a deviant person among them, then the deviant person is rejected. In suicidal behaviour we see that when a family member is rejected, after all sanctions have failed to change his behaviour, then suicide occurs. Suicide and alcoholism are often linked together (Appleby 1992; Frances and Borg 1993; Henriksson *et al.* 1993; Lepine, Chignon and Teherani 1993; Sonneck and Wagner 1996) and we see a common systemic process of escalating distress.

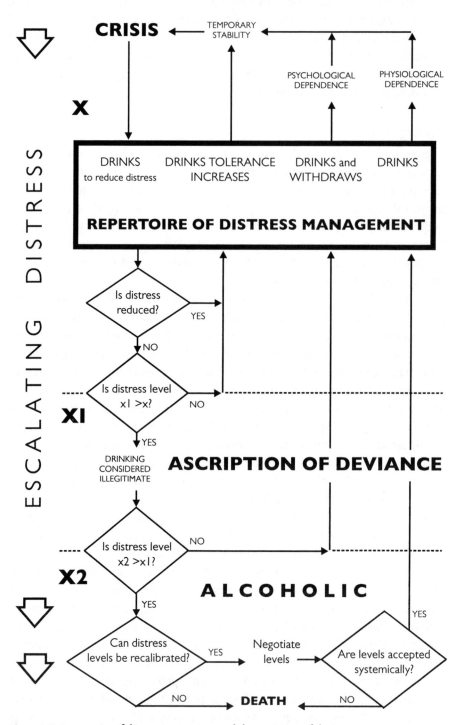

Figure 5.2 A repertoire of distress management and the ascription of deviance

The cycle of drinking in the management of distress

As individuals we negotiate within ourselves the tolerances for healthy functioning such that as organic systems we remain intact. These tolerances are also negotiated in performance with others. In Figure 5.2 we see a model of distress management that is built upon the cycle of distress management previously found in suicidal behaviour (Aldridge 1998). I am assuming that drinking is self-damaging yet serves a performative purpose within nested social contexts of intimate relationship, family and community. The point chosen to start this cycle is that of a system facing a crisis. I am using system here to refer to a small group of intimate others in relationship. It could refer in some cases to an individual alone as a self-enclosed system. This is rarely the case. Drinkers have friends or, if not friends, social workers. Something happens. A life event occurs. This event can be a change in mood, a disappointment, the recurrence of pain or an argument. Whatever, something happens that constitutes an 'event' for those intimates. In Batesonian terms there is 'news of difference' (Bateson 1972, 1978). There is a comparison between what is and an idealized situation. While this process is 'social', it is the comparison that also makes it 'individual', involving thoughts and feelings, psychology and physiology. As we see in suicidal behaviour in families, family members may share similar constructions of meaning but there are individual constitutive rules regarding the interpretations of those constructs.

Thresholds of distress are threatened (see section X in Fig. 5.2). The drinker takes a drink to reduce his distress, or when he takes the drink his partner calms down knowing everything will be OK. The crisis is over. Distress is reduced. Stability is maintained. Everything is fine. This is a simple homeostatic loop (Beer 1975) as we see in section X of Figure 5.2. Distress is performed and alleviated. We have a repertoire of distress management in a relational context that becomes embodied in one person. This embodiment literally entails a change in the tolerance of alcohol. There is a physiological consequence of personal and social acts. Tolerance is suitably ambiguous here, as it implies both a physical tolerance and a tolerance of such behaviour within a relationship. It may sound strange but it can literally be in some instances that 'I take a drink and you calm down'. We take the logic of relational actions into our own bodies. The same process has been demonstrated in the management of blood sugar levels in children during episodes of family stress (Minuchin 1974; Minuchin *et al.* 1975). Habits are literally formed, they achieve a material reality, a *habitus*.

Should distress not be reduced then an alternative strategy from the repertoire of distress management may be used (see level X1, Figure 5.2). For the drinker this may be more drinking, going on a 'binge' away from the relationship or having a row. He withdraws. His partner withdraws. Distance occurs in the relationship. At this stage his drinking behaviour becomes labelled as deviant. If, however, overall distress is reduced by this constellation of drinking behaviours, whether in himself or within his family, then we have the situation set for dependence. In the medical and psychological literature this will be seen as an individual psychological dependence. If however we take a systemic perspective, the other is as dependent as the drinker is on his drinking. Nevertheless, the situation is deemed to be getting 'out of control'. Like tolerance, dependence is suitably ambiguous. It is not simply that the drinker becomes dependent upon alcohol, his intimates become dependent upon his resolving their mutual distress.

In systemic terms, the premises by which the system maintains its integrity are becoming challenged. System refers to the individual drinker and those with whom he shares his life, but this 'system' also belongs to a wider eco-system of family, friends and environment. A subset of such premises will be concerned with the management of distress and how that distress can be controlled. An axiom of a systems perspective is that no one part can have unilateral control over the whole. Bateson describes that such a belief in 'control' is the essential epistemological fallacy of the alcoholic (Bateson 1972). If this is so, then it is the epistemological fallacy of medical science and of the postmodern if it locates control in the individual and loses its ecological understanding.

If distress continues or further crises occur and drinking itself becomes one of those crises, then the drinker and his family attempt to accommodate a higher level of distress. (Distress at X2 in Figure 5.2 is greater than at X and X1). When this occurs a family with a member who becomes symptomatic to maintain family stability becomes a family system with a necessarily symptomatic member. The deviant drinker becomes labelled as an alcoholic. Not only is the repertoire of distress management extended, but the initial thresholds of distress are altered. The system returns to a stable state but that state is altered and the alcoholic becomes physiologically dependent. It is here that we have the logical basis, in medical terms, for the ascription of disease. It is also the end point in the process of somatization. The danger is that once the arbiter of distress, the alcoholic, becomes the cause of distress and embodies the distress of those with whom he lives, then his repertoire of distress management, that has now become monolithically drinking, will kill him. He drinks himself to death. As Greco (1998a) writes:

A diseased state is also regulated by norms, though these are different from healthy ones and inferior to them, in fact, they leave the organism a smaller margin of tolerance for the inconsistencies of the environment. It is plausible to suggest, of course, that what we *call* illness, what we *collectively* recognise as such, is what deviates from a given range of social norms which varies across cultures. (Greco 1998a, p.241)

An appropriate treatment strategy would appear to be to introduce a repertoire of distress management that offers an alternative to drowning his and others sorrows and this must be delivered within a social context. Drinking becomes both the means of presenting distress and the means of resolving distress, temporarily. By taking a medical, disease perspective, rather than a metaphoric perspective, then the practitioner is colluding with the material presentation of distress and ignoring the long-term problem. Medication for the treatment of alcoholism is simply a short-term resolution of a problem that maintains the problem in the long term. The treatment becomes part of the same strategy because it participates in the same misguided solution of veiling the awareness necessary for change. We see the same pattern repeated in the treatment of other somatic presentations of distress like anorexia nervosa and repetitions of deliberate self-harm when the purpose of the malady is unrecognized within the ecology that it maintains (Aldridge 1998). Discovering what that purpose in life is and transcending current meanings to achieve a new awareness of life are precisely what the spiritual endeavour is concerned with.

Alcoholics Anonymous

So far we have seen that alcoholism is the embodiment of distress. The sufferer becomes isolated from those contexts where a new identity can be performed and which will offer her means for transcending current understandings. If spirituality is the search for meaning and purpose and transcending the current situation, then she is in spiritual need. As we saw in the chapter on religion, the context for the performance of new meanings is through social contact. Therefore, any recovery will need to take place with others. This spiritual awakening through mutual contact was a fundamental idea in the beginning of Alcoholics Anonymous.

In the early stages of the movement that was to become Alcoholics Anonymous the founders were in a dilemma. The Oxford Movement in which they were involved had provided a theological perspective by which the sinner could be saved. Yet, this perspective was deemed to be too religious, too churchy (Kurtz 1979). It emphasized God, with a capital G, and was aggressively evangelical and moralistic. In the USA in the early 1930s such a perspective was not attractive to the derelicts on skid row or the drinkers in the suburbs. Although a spiritual perspective, respecting that alcoholics are powerless and their lives had become unmanageable and only God could restore them to sanity, were the first two steps to recovery, a religious perspective was vigorously denied. Fellowship was emphasized but an organized religion was taken to be unattractive to possible recruits and as an affront to some Catholics.

Alcoholics had also had enough of being preached at by the temperance movement and felt themselves as being sick not sinners, hence the welcoming of alcoholism as being an allergy, like a disease, and a mental obsession. Churches were seen to have failed them and spiritual experience gained through personal revelation and fellowship provided an open alternative. However, even the mention of God in the first three steps to recovery of Alcoholics Anonymous was to be too much and God became a 'Power greater than ourselves' and 'God as we understand him'. This seems like a prescience of what has since happened within the field of new religious movements where god is thrown out in favour of greater power. It is also a rejection of the dogmatism of 'God said' and an authoritarian approach that religions have attempted to maintain and which science too had rejected. Nevertheless, a spiritual perspective emphasizing a power greater than the individual was the first step to recovery. 'God', as each individual understood him as a higher power, was to return the drinker to sanity, even though this higher power was still a gendered reality.

A gesture of humility

Initially recognizing this power meant going down on one's knees to pray. It was also a legacy of the evangelical church background and a sign of repentance. For those who did not know what the power greater than themselves was or, indeed, how to pray, this was the first step. To an increasingly sophisticated psychologized culture this appeared an unnecessary humiliation, and so it was in the movement itself. But the early days of Alcoholics Anonymous contain stories of how people were vigorously encouraged to get down on their knees. Literally here is the crux of the matter. If alcoholism is the somatization of distress and an arrogant belief in self-control, a self-control that cannot be maintained, the show of humility by getting down on one's knees is the necessary first step. If embodiment is important for communication to others and, as importantly, as a sign of accept-ance that we make within ourselves, then this was literally the first *movement* to recovery: not the first thought, not the first feeling, but the initial gesture like being pushed off a cliff.

While we are highly verbal beings who celebrate the complexities of a communicative culture, we cannot deny the power of gesture. Indeed, for the somatic presentation of distress, then a bodily gesture is absolutely symmetrical to that presentation. Like meets like. We do still speak, in English language cultures, of events that literally bring us to our knees. If we have the embodiment of distress, in this move onto the knees, we also have the embodiment of humility, the submission before a greater power. All spiritual traditions have emphasized this essential posture for prayer and particularly in meditation. While we may think of meditation as specifically control over the mind, and thereby control over the body, the basis of most practices is initially a specifically adopted posture. Unfortunately in modern cultures a show of humility in gesture is often con-stitutively interpreted as an humiliation, thereby losing a potential benefit. Getting down on one's knees before a personally recognized higher power or

God as understood by the drinker is a significant change from getting down on the knees before an authoritarian church hierarchy. It is certainly preferable to falling down in the gutter.

Recognition of imperfection

The third step on the road to recovery was that the founders of the movement 'Made a decision to turn our will and our lives over to the care of God' (Kurtz 1979), to which was added later the tag 'as we understood him' (Bergmark 1998; Kurtz 1979). If the alcoholic was no longer to be in control of his life, there had to be some source to which he could turn. The use of God was to feature in a further four of the twelve steps to recovery that included confession of wrongdoing, repentance, supplication and submission. These were to lead to the declaration in the twelfth step that reaffirmed the spiritual awakening brought about by these steps and that this message was to be carried further to other alcoholics. I shall return to this message of awakening later. Essentially, the recognition of god, liberally interpreted as representing a higher power, identifies a relationship between the subjective and the objective. There is an awareness of the individual and the universal as ideal, and therefore a knowledge of difference. Where this source is located, god within or god without, is individually interpreted according to the world view of the participant. In essence it allows the alcoholic to be imperfect and accepted. Only god is perfect. It also allows the alcoholic to escape the ethnic identity of religion and emphasizes the possibility of an individualized spirituality.

Two steps to recovery were originally formulated as 'Made a searching and fearless moral inventory of ourselves' and 'Continued to take personal inventory and when we were wrong admitted it' (Kurtz 1979). The 'moral' from moral inventory has since been dropped, but the initial impulse was to admit to what had been done wrong and where the alcoholic had been fooling himself and others. This was a merciless confrontation, but necessary. However, self-confrontation was also linked to another step that demanded the alcoholic make amends where possible, except when to do so would injure themselves or others. So while there is a personal culpability, an ethic, this is also related to acts that must be performed as reparation, and the vehicle for this is a higher power. This is also a restoration of relationship and a release from isolation. The moral is the social and reparation is a return to a social world away from seclusion.

The message of awakening

'The telling of personal experience – *internal* personal experience – laid the foundation for saving identification. The antidote for the deep symptom of denial was *identification* marked by open and undemanding narration infused with profound honesty about personal weakness' (Kurtz 1979).

We read in Chapter 1 that narrative is the centre of a performed identity. Language is important for the way in which we author our identities and the language of spirituality enhances the repertoires of healing vocabularies that we have by transforming and transcending understandings. A vocabulary that includes hope, transcendence, forgiveness and grace will be important in how we author our identity. Identities are authored through action and involvement with others. As we see in the citation above, narration based on the twelve steps to recovery is a powerful antidote to the denial of the alcoholic. It offers a means of identification but discerning the appropriate vocabulary for that identification which was important in the early days, just as we have to be careful in formulating a vocabulary of healing today. Gone are the days of 'God said' and a religious authority. Emphasizing 'God as we understand him' by Alcoholics Anonymous was the important postmodern step in emphasizing a subjective awareness. This was not only the alcoholic as 'Not-God' as Kurtz says, but also an identity that was 'Not-Ethnic' and 'Not-Christian' or 'Not-Islam'. It is a move away from the 'hatred machines' of organized religion (Cupitt 1997) to a performed identity, temporary and with others who too have suffered.

Bill Wilson, as a founder of Alcoholics Anonymous, in trying to discern how the programme worked, hit upon the idea that it was the telling of the story by sober alcoholics which was central to the process of recovery. Not only do stories convey information that something has happened, the very act of narrating has a healing potential. While the focus of the narration is often on the listeners' experience, what we have in Alcoholics Anonymous is the idea that the telling of the tale is primary. The telling of the tale, as testimony, is the healing for the teller. In traditional religious terms this was simply 'I was lost and now I am found'. In the evangelical church movement, the idea of testimony was to express just that.

Testimonies are personal narratives told publicly. They are narratives that have to be witnessed, and witnessing a narrative was a significant part of the non-orthodox church movements. There is a personal and a relational element present. When the narrative is repeated, and it is expected that the personal narrative is repeated in public settings, it is the responsibility of those present to scrutinize that narrative and remind the narrator if her public testimony deviates from the truth as they know it. So while a personal narrative is expressed, the process of confrontation takes place if the teller tries to put a gloss on that narrative other than the truth as experienced. This provides the important location of narrative within a social context and presents the context for an improvised reality bounded by a commonality of understanding.

Salvation in the telling

Repeating her own story was to become the salvation for the former drunk that kept her sober. This is a significant turnaround from the narrative experience as we know it today. The therapeutic effect in Alcoholics Anonymous is also for the teller, not solely the listener. The listener might hear the call and through a divine intervention respond. For the teller, the giving away of his spiritual knowledge keeps him dry. We read in Kurtz (1979) that some drinkers were astounded when visitors recounted their stories of drink and despair, telling them they had the answer and then going away without offering any pat solution. It was when the listener wanted the answer that he was given it. The conditions were offered but it was necessary for the impulse for change to come from the drinker himself. This was the beginning of the awakening.

In many counselling approaches, in psychotherapy and for most health-care professionals, the activity of skilled listening is emphasized. We also have within qualitative research a growing interest in narrative methods. However, these approaches always place the emphasis on the listener. It is the listener that is the healer; the listener, as researcher, that interprets and categorizes. The listener retains power. However, in testimony, it is the teller who retains the power in the telling; not a personal power, but a spiritual power that must be continually revived through telling unless she fall sick again. While we have emphasized listening skills in counselling, we have missed a major point. It is the skills of the teller, the person who comes in need, that are important, and how we offer the context for the telling of his tale, the relationship that holds this telling.

We saw the same process in the ward of a psychiatric hospital where patients were said to be suicidal and through the letters of women who had been deliberately harming themselves (Aldridge 1998). When they were allowed to make their own testimonies, and testimonies that were witnessed by a researcher rather than by a therapist, then the suicidal behaviour was reduced. My arrogance as researcher was to believe that my role as listener, not even as a therapist, helped these women. Indeed, unexplainably at the time, when neutral listening was introduced as a therapeutic strategy, it failed. Ross and Mckay (1979) had found the same inexplicable pattern earlier. Once allowing a story to be narrated was allowed, then a therapeutic benefit was achieved. Maybe we have made a serious mistake in theory regarding therapy by believing that it is our listening skills that have to be honed, whereas it is simply allowing the teller to tell her tale to a listener without being judged that is important.

The emphasis is placed on the narrator. Repeating a successful tale maintains the positive process, just as we know that repeating a tale of disaster without resolution is at the heart of the litanies of pain and depression we hear in everyday practice. In addition, by changing the context of listening to research and *not* therapy, then there is a change in the power relationship. For my research, the teller was in control of a valuable narrative, her testimony. In a therapeutic context, she was always asking for help, embodying the distress and rehearsing that distress which made her sick and separate, reflecting her loss of power in the relationship. In a research context there was a shift in the balance of that power; no testimony, no data, no PhD.

If we recall Eva in Chapter 1, she had a story to tell about what her problem was regarding her loss of God. We accepted the loss of her husband. We understood that she was depressed. We readily categorized her as suicidal and provisionally categorized her as mentally ill. It was only when her story was really heard, when she was allowed to tell it fully, that she began to find the relief which she had sought. It is to my chagrin that I regarded this as a process of listening when really it was the process of telling that brought about the change. A context was offered where she could tell what had to be told, but that is the very least that we can do as practitioners. The therapeutic effect, the healing, did not lie in my hands. It was in her testimony, that had to be witnessed, where a clearing appeared in the forest of distress such that change could take place.

The question remains about how we handicap others from achieving their own healing through restricting the options for telling and relating. Maybe the various anecdotes that we hear about success in complementary therapies is actually in the recounting of the story of healing. If this is so, then the same will apply to any medical encounter. The efficacy lies in the relating of recovery. This does not deny the medical intervention as part of the process but that process is completed by allowing the recovery to be related in the language of the patient according to her criteria in her own time. This is not the same as taking time to listen in the preliminary consultations where diagnosis takes place, where tales of illness are told and medicines prescribed. This is taking time to listen to recovery and what is being done about it. The process of healing requires its narrative completion as testimonial. A testimonial has to be witnessed and this is perhaps where we see the benefit of the varying Church health-care initiatives in that not only do they promote access to welfare, but also provide witness to testimonial through fellowship.

To whom the tale is told

If we return to the early Alcoholics Anonymous movement we also see that it was not professional counsellors who were important but former drunks telling their tales. This has ramifications for the democratization of health-care delivery where self-care health groups are providing the basis for successful community endeav-ours in the field of chronic illness. It is tales of spiritual awakening and recovery told by former sufferers that are central to healing and recovery in Alcoholics Anonymous. These very elements are discarded in the process of professionalization of health-care. The evidence of the anecdote heals the teller, as giver, and inspires the receiver, yet in modern medicine fails to count as evidence. Testimony assumes veracity. We have to trust each other in the use of words and to do this we also need a witness. Personal accounts are witnessed by others which lends them veracity. Our lives are lived and performed with others. When we discount the anecdotal we are not only throwing out the process of healing but saying that we belong to a community of liars.

Return to the subject

As we read in Chapter 1, modern society appears to be dehumanizing because it fails to grasp the emotional responses necessary for 'being for the other'. Modernity is based upon control, with a distance placed between the observer and events. In a socially responsible healing culture, this distance must be replaced. We are literally being asked to 'be there' by the other and to be there in a sensual relationship that will entail a lived body. It is this loss of the concept of 'other', loss of the 'drunk' or the 'deviant', the dissolution of a dualism, that is central to spiritual understandings; hence the Christian invocation, though we are many, we are one body (Aldridge 1987c). We promote a sense of unity when we and the other become one.

In a postmodern world where health is the presentation of self then we have the formula for alienation from an inner identity. A performed identity, denied access to a true self, when performed at the interface of a legitimating public, or perhaps better expressed as with a legitimating public, is a process of objectification. We lose the subject as identity. We lose sight of what we are as a potential to be transformed. Therefore, no matter how fit, healthy, successful or perfect we appear, something is lacking. In the process of narration, of offering testimony, we have a reflection on the self as it was and the opportunity to compare then and now. The achievement of this new identity is brought about by a spiritual awakening, through inspiration. A new identity is performed that is always imperfect and constantly being improvised. Alcoholics take things one day at a time.

We have also the capacity to be private. We perform a narrative with ourselves that is reflective. In doing so we can engage in the process of prayer, as telling and meditation, as listening. These processes have both been the sources of healing as we will see in the next chapter. In Alcoholics Anonymous a 'Serenity prayer' is often used (Steffen 1993). This prayer asks that 'God grant us the serenity to accept the things that we cannot change, courage to change the things that we can, and wisdom to know the difference' (quoted in Bateson 1972). Effectively breaking the cycle of control, this prayer dissuades us from seeking to influence everything yet retains a limited personal agency. Dossey (1993) writes that the underlying desire for total personal, conscious control and responsibility in health is frequently a narcissistic desire for power (p.67). The trick is being able to know the difference between what can be influenced and what cannot, as the prayer for serenity entreats, and that entails consciousness. By using prayer, it is possible to invoke the consciousness that brings knowledge and the impulse towards unity. Thus we have transcendence and the basis of spirituality. What we also learn from Alcoholics Anonymous is that we cannot do it alone, we need a friend; not a therapist, a friend.

Coda

The history of Alcoholics Anonymous mirrors the modern history of complementary medicines in some ways. Alcoholics Anonymous is predominantly a lay movement that sought to gain validity and in its search for validity attempted to adopt a medical language and demanded that alcoholism be identified as a disease. It is a warning to many unconventional therapies that would be adopted into the field of conventional medical practices.

Alcoholics Anonymous was based on an individual spiritual awakening recognizing God, as the individual understood god, as an ultimate power. To achieve recovery, the drinker had to get down on her knees, acknowledge god from her own subjective viewpoint, repent and repair her wrongdoing. To retain her sobriety she had to reflect upon her own imperfection, tell others how low she had sunk and how she had been saved through an awareness of god in her life. Once sober, she was expected to maintain her own sobriety by telling other drunks what had happened to her. By giving away what she had gained, she could retain sobriety and offer other drinkers a chance to realize the same condition. Rather than this being a moral viewpoint of a large-scale doctrinal system, it is an ethic, a way of life done day by day with people who understand through experience. Rather than seeking to change the other through personal power, it is an emphasis on relationship that offers the other the possibility to achieve awareness. Admitting the pragmatic benefits of such an approach, drunks dried out and stopped drinking, one day at a time. This means regular attendance at Alcoholics Anonymous meetings and we cannot discount the social nature of such gatherings offering stable relationships modelling sobriety as we saw in Chapter 3.

Medicine, seeing the benefits, adopted the programme to cure alcoholism. This assumption of cure invalidates all that Alcoholics Anonymous stands for. The basis for the drinker is that there is no cure. He is imperfect. That is the meaning and the purpose of the malady, to understand imperfection and temporality in relation to perfection and eternity. He understands his reliance upon a higher power. Even if he does not drink, he is always open to some other failing. There is no cure for being human and fallible. Yet, he lives his life as whole understanding the continuing need for the spiritual, accepting that there are some things he can change, things that he cannot, praying he will know the difference; what we may regard as the normal human condition. If, as Alcoholics Anonymous asserts, the alcoholic becomes so because he denies the spiritual and demands absolute control over his emotions, then by denying the spiritual aspects of recovery and emphasizing personal control scientific medicine is proposing the very cycle of pathology that maintains the addiction. By substituting an alternative substance and calling it medication, little is changed. The same strategy is maintained for alleviating distress.

What scientific medicine does in trying to understand such an approach is to take on the parts that it can understand. First, out goes God as a subjective understanding. God belongs to religion and not science. However, a greater power is tolerable as a concept, if such a power is interpreted as energy. The problem remains that such energy is elusive to measurement and in healing seems to deny physical laws of distance (Dossey 1982, 1993). Out goes the 'kneeling' part of submission as it is humiliating and unseemly for the autonomous individual, even if he is a drunk and has 'hit bottom'. An idealized view of being human is maintained that elevates perfection, the very opposite of the humility that we have seen is necessary incorporating the acceptance of imperfection and limitation. Furthermore, the 'one day at a time' perspective is ignored. If treatment outcomes are considered as evidence of efficacy for a treatment programme and as a basis for funding, then who is going to devise a follow-up study that makes sense on a one day at a time basis? But, to be congruent to the original treatment philosophy it would need to be so. Part of the efficacy of Alcoholics Anonymous is in the modesty of the claims.

The social side of reparation and confession is accepted because it fits in with a confessional technology of psychotherapy and counselling. Telling stories about being drunk and subsequent recovery is acceptable but locates the healing abilities in the professional listener alone. Treatment institutions then insist, to make everything legitimate, that these listeners are trained and appropriately licensed. I am not arguing against licensing or training, simply that the point is being missed by locating the healing abilities in the listener alone. In the Alcoholics Anonymous approach, it is the tellers, the former drinkers licensed through suffering, that maintain healing in themselves. The power balance in Alcoholics Anonymous is the fellow drinker now dry having to tell his testimony to maintain sobriety in the hope that the listener will hear his own call as a mutual sufferer, to that of the skilled counsellor, listening and categorizing what he is told by a sick or deviant other. First the source of healing is discarded and then the nature of the relationship as the location for that healing.

Epistemology and healing

There is no magic by which one person heals the other. There is a change in consciousness that brings about recovery on behalf of the person who submits and prays. All she can do is tell her story to the other, but it is always for her own benefit first. Those who calls themselves spiritual healers may indeed be practising healing, but it is for their own salvation. This talk of healing may lead the patient to find her own way anew and experience healing within herself, but then who is the healer? If the practice of religion is primarily concerned with the exercise of power, then religious healing will simply reflect that moral imperative to restore order and convention in the identified 'sick' other.

A spiritual perspective claims no such power and is concerned with an individual ethic as consciousness of a higher self, or seeing oneself as related to the universal. Illness is potentially also an impulse that returns us to consciousness. Suffering has its purpose. I am not here advocating a lifelong gratitude to viruses and bacteria, rather that even through the trials and tribulations of being an organism alive in a living world, the seething plethora of creation, we regain what it is to have human consciousness.

If being for the other is seen as a part of healing, then we are all surely potentially a healing context. It is the minimal requirement of being human that we are available for others. If the healer considers herself as the source of healing rather than the conditions, or part of the context, then she is committing the epistemological fallacy of the alcoholic, she is becoming 'god'. Finally, if health is a performed identity that is creative, then the source of that creativity will need to be continuously sought. Others may play a part in the mutual performance but to identify them as the source of healing is to miss the point.

At the heart of this approach is a simple gesture of kneeling; an initiatory impulse of prayer and admittance that there is another power greater than one's own. This takes place in relationship with fellow sufferers and is repeated within a social context that models sobriety. We all need a friend. Its claims are limited and modest, to stop drinking one day at a time. The basis of this is described as a spiritual awakening. We have then elements of the physical, psychological, social and spiritual together.

6

Prayer and healing

If you can't handle your feelings, how can you avoid harming your spirit? If you can't control your emotions, but nevertheless try to stop yourself following them, you will harm yourself twice over. Those who do this double injury to themselves are not counted amongst those with long life. (Chang Tzu in Palmer 1996)

Thus far you have harmonized with your body, having the usual nine apertures, and you have not been struck midway through life with blindness or deafness, lameness nor any deformity, so in comparison to many you are fortunate. So why do you wander around grumbling about Heaven? Be gone, Sir! (Chang Tzu in Palmer 1996)

We read in the last chapter that by using prayer, it is possible to invoke the consciousness that brings knowledge. Thus we have transcendence and the basis of spirituality seen in Chapter 2. Consciousness is promoted by a posture, in this latter example, kneeling. Something is done, one small gesture, but a gesture in a chain of possibilities. It is located within a personal context of abject suffering and a relational context of caring and mutual disclosure. The sufferer has hit bottom. A friend helps. A story is told. Meanings and purposes are realized anew and there is an understanding of a unifying consciousness, a higher power, or god. Whatever that name is, it is appropriate, but consciousness is prior to naming. A simple act in a context of caring promotes the realization of an ecology of ideas.

A central requirement is that a personal sense of self is abandoned and a higher power acknowledged. We find our niche in the total ecology, an ecology that includes ideas, emotions, activities and a change in attitude. We become whole, healed, temporarily. Disclosure, the telling of a personal narrative both by the drinker now dry to maintain his dryness and the drinker who has reached bottom is an important step. This abandoning of self and the act of disclosure is central to the act of prayer. In a series of studies by Pennebaker (Dienstfrey 1999a), writing as disclosure of distressing experiences is seen to have health-care benefits. Telling is also disclosure. The acts of writing and telling are active and dynamic; not the narrative but the narrating, not the prayer but the praying.

In religious traditions, this telling to a god or higher power is called prayer. It may include a petition on behalf of oneself or for another asking for restoration or reparation. There are prayers that the sick make to restore health and prayers that others make on behalf of the sick that they be made well. Some prayers are concerned with forgiveness of the self or for others. Some prayers are concerned with saying how bad the world is, how awful we have been treated and that this situation is recognized and remediated. Some prayers are concerned with expressing gratitude to a higher power, others with praising the bounties of life and nature. Prayer then is an expressive form. As an expressive form it may also use utterances rather than words. In this way, the petitioner does not have to be concerned with either an elegance of language or a sophisticated and extended vocabulary. Prayers may take the form of movements, gestures and ecstatic outbursts, hence the varying forms of religious expression according to the cultures and the times in which they are necessary.

Yet another range of prayers is concerned with being quiet and contemplative. These are meditative prayers (see Table 6.1). There are no fixed boundaries and the person praying may move from contemplation to active expression and back to quiet contemplation again.

Table 6.1 Forms of prayer and their content	
Meditative prayer	A time spent in reflecting upon the divine with the intent of achieving a unified presence such that there is no separation. Sometimes described as resting in the arms of God. The person praying is listening and experiencing unity as a presence.
Intercessory prayer	The person praying talks to the divine using his or her own words. The prayer may include asking for help in decision making, requesting the resolution of specific problems and petitioning for the relief of suffering, but could be just as well concerned with praise, thanksgiving or worship.
	These are purposive prayers that vary in their specificity and degree of formality. Such prayers are usually seen in reports of spiritual and religious healing where specific health-care outcomes are offered as petitions.
Liturgical prayer	Each religion has formalized prayers with approved texts to support them. These prayers are incorporated within a liturgical structure and may be accompanied by specific injunctions to kneel, stand, extend the hands or lie prostrate.
	These are ritualized forms of prayer. Such rituals may include formal periods of intercessory prayer for the sick. Church healing services for the sick may be ritualized and also include sessions where spontaneous intercessory prayer can take place.

Prayers may also be conducted privately alone, in small groups, in public or collectively as a congregation. The essence of these approaches is that the person praying loses herself before a higher power or experience of the divine that some call 'God' such that they are merged. This is the realization of unity that is sought. Sincerity of prayer, rather than form, is considered to be paramount and spoken forms and gestures are considered to be efficacious in that they make thoughts concrete. Words prayed without thought are considered to be vain repetitions (Khan 1974). These prayers can be spoken out loud or silently invoked. At its essence, prayer is to be in the presence of the divine. To reach some stages of prayer requires teaching, instruction or guidance.

Forms of prayer

As we saw in earlier chapters, there are varying definitions of spirituality, religion and health and these are realized in differing forms. The same can be said of prayer. Nevertheless, there are discernible commonalities to prayer. At the risk of being unnecessarily coarse I shall try and reduce these varying prayer forms to three types: meditative prayer, intercessory prayer and liturgical prayer (see Table 6.1).

In terms of healing prayers, intercessory prayer is perhaps used most often as we will see below. In a study of clergy using prayer as pastoral care with patients in hospital, it is a spontaneous intercessory form of prayer that is used predominantly (VandeCreek 1998). In the previous chapter, praying for the serenity to accept the things that cannot be changed, the courage to change the things that can be changed, and the wisdom to know the difference is an important part of maintaining sobriety. While this is an intercession, it is not a simple plea for healing or a cure. Within it is an intercession for discernment and, thereby, knowledge.

An accompaniment to intercessory prayers may include the gesture of a laying on of hands. This is symbolic of the divine reaching out to the petitioner to heal, in the sense of making whole, as a sacrament of healing. The laying on of hands as intercession combined with prayers has been incorporated in Church healing movements (Aldridge 1987c; Csordas 1997; Griffith 1983). The significance of the sacrament of the laying on of hands is as a sacred reality (Csordas 1983) and not to be equated, as by some writers, with the therapeutic touch of the doctor as a secular reality. Sickness when placed in the hands of a divine authority releases the patients to a new form of living and integration within a community. As in Alcoholics Anonymous, we see the preservation of an ecology, the individual is healed within a community. Neither is prior.

Hand healing, however, has also acquired a meaning associated with healing touch and the transference of energies (Engebretson 1996; Wuthnow 1997). It is referred to as a form of spiritual healing (Wirth 1993) that we will see later is used in general medical practice with some success for the treatment of chronic problems (Brown and Sheldon 1989; Dixon 1998). Solfin (1984) calls these approaches, including spiritual healing, 'mental healing', as the situation is characterized by a mental intention to help or heal.

Magaletta and Brawer (1998) contend that prayer is a central organizing principle in most religions, like Schmied (1998) who sees prayer as the activation of religion and McKinney and McKinney (1999), who regard prayer as the essence of religion (see Table 6.2). Yet prayer also assumes a dispositional character, as if it were a style of living (Magaletta and Brawer 1998) and in no way exceptional (Dossey 1993). It is also relational, either described as a conversational dialogue (Cavanaugh 1994; McKinney and McKinney 1999), as awareness of a presence (Khan 1974), as an invitation to heal (Magaletta and Brawer 1998), or an intention to seek healing (Magaletta and Brawer 1998). As there are varying religious forms, then prayer too will alter its form, purpose and content, which has proved to be a confounding factor in spiritual healing research using prayer as a treatment strategy.

Mike

Mike knew he was dying. His doctor had told him, his body had told him and the priest came to visit. The priest coming to visit emphasized how sad Mike's plight had become as he was no churchgoer. Indeed, his life had been one of rebellion and delinquency by his own admission. But in recent years he had married, held down a job, started a family and was buying a house. Life had changed for the better in terms of what he wanted.

His daughter was eighteen months old when Mike was first diagnosed with cancer. He became increasingly agitated, pacing the house and picking arguments aggressively with friends, neighbours and people in the supermarket. A style of life that he thought he had left behind began to surface again. He was dis-contented. Literally the content of his life that was satisfying was being lost. Even his appearance was changing to one he had left behind. His now hairless head, as the result of chemotherapy, reminded him of his head once shaven in defiance.

A family friend of Mike's asked a local priest to visit to see if he could be counselled. The local priest then asked me to intervene as he thought that relaxation and meditation techniques were perhaps more appropriate.

On visiting Mike and his family it was quickly apparent that Mike was becoming desperate in that nobody was talking to him about dying. He knew that things were serious because both a priest and a psychologist came to his home to visit. It became a joke in a local church that you knew if you were really ill or not if your name was mentioned in intercessory prayers for the sick. If you had a subsequent home visit, then things were going downhill fast.

Table 6.2 Prayer definitions

Definitions	Author
Prayer is that for religion, what thinking is for philosophy … the activation of religion in its proper sense. (p.116)	Schmied quoting Novalis and Thomas Aquinas (1998)
[Prayer is] every kind of inward communion or conversation with the power recognised as divine… Prayer in this wide sense is the very soul and essence of religion. (p.280)	McKinney and McKinney quoting William James (1999)
Prayer is not an innovation, it is a process of remembering who we really are and how we are related. From this point of view, there is a good reason to rid prayer of its aura that it is some rare state we enter only on certain occasions. If the unity it connotes is not the exception but the rule, there should be no celestial halo surrounding prayer. (p.114)	Dossey (1993)
They [conservative theologians] might strengthen their concept of prayer by defining the subconscious as a way station for burdens on the way to and from God. Certainly they would agree that the conscious end of the dialogue, where problems and answers are articulated in words, is identical with classical prayer, unless prayer is held to require magical incantations of specific words and names. (p.250)	Cavanaugh (1994)
Prayer is in reality the contemplation of God's presence…and it is considering oneself as nothing before Him, and placing the wish which stands before one's personality before the Almighty. (p.87)	Khan (1974)
'The divine agent assumption' assumes that prayer in therapy invites a Higher Power to actively engage in the healing process. (p.322) Besides being operationalized as a behaviour, prayer can also be defined as a dispositional state, a way of living, or an approach to life. (p.323) Prayer may be the client's ongoing effort to seek healing from emotional and/or physical distress, or it may occur as the result of a prescriptive or encouraging suggestion given by the therapist. (p.323)	Magaletta and Brawer (1998)

He knew he had little time to live, from what he had been told, but nobody was talking to him about how to die. He was so desperate, he said, that he would pray if he knew how! He had not told this to his priest as it was embarrassing to have to admit that it was not something which he had ever done before. He also did not want 'the full Church treatment', meaning by this that the words and sacraments and all the piety of expression would have been too strange; not to mention the well-meaning visitors anxious to help. This reflects the early years of Alcoholics Anonymous that we saw in the previous chapter, where an approach which was too 'churchy' was rejected.

What also emerged was that he thought of prayer as essentially a childish activity since every time he came to consider praying he found himself ready to ask like a child to a father. That his father was abusive and had rejected him was a significant factor in preventing his prayer. Becoming an adult man, no longer under the dominance of his father, had been a major struggle for him. To ask him to return to such a stage of submission was psychologically incompatible. Through the use of guided imagery and meditation (Aldridge 1987c) it was possible to help him find a way to contemplate that was satisfactory to his needs and which helped him also to forgive his father.

He became less agitated and his family life improved. His wife became less distressed, his daughter enjoyed having her father to play with at home and the wider family became involved. He died within five weeks of first being contacted.

There we have the problem of healing prayer and outcomes research if we take a restricted perspective on prayer and healing efficacy. People die. As my medical colleagues said, 'It [prayer] doesn't work.' Mike died. As the centuries reveal, some people remain sick despite prayer (McCullough 1995).

Yet, something changed about him that was evident in what he did, improved the quality of his immediate family life and sufficiently eased his last few weeks alive, meeting some of his psychological and spiritual needs. There was understanding and reconciliation and surely these are valuable factors in health care for the survivors as well as the identified sufferer (Aldridge 1987a, 1987b, 1987d; Holt, Houg and Romano 1999). Survivors suffer too and need relief. Family members need to discuss dealing with the hurts, angers and conflicts they have experienced with each other (Aponte 1998; Hargrave and Sells 1997; Walrond-Skinner 1998). The time before death can be used to bring old conflicts to a close, to say goodbye and seek forgiveness from others, to express love and gratitude for the gifts of a life (Mermann 1992), although this depends upon the maturity of those involved (Pingleton 1997). Forgiveness is a central feature in religion and we are becoming increasingly aware of its role in a healing ecology for practitioners as well as the patient and caregivers (Aponte 1998; Canale *et al.* 1996; Ferch 1998; Pollard *et al.* 1998).

Prayer has been used over the centuries to promote a sense of union with the divine, to gain access to a spiritual power and to seek nourishment for the soul. Yet, major religions have warned that this activity is not a matter simply of cause and effect. The process of prayer is not one of self-seeking, or of asking in a concentrated manner that a bounty will necessarily ensue. Prayer is a matter of self-dedication and remembering where we belong in a greater unity.

McCullough (1995) reminds us that in the Christian Bible there are stories where people actually become worse through prayer. Like the drinker in the previous chapter, we have to go through the dark night of the soul and reach rock bottom: 'Thus, some benefits of prayer may materialise only after life has become considerably worse than it was before praying' (McCullough 1995, p.16). Not a great consolation for those seeking a direct correlation between prayer and health outcomes and certainly less than encouraging for those promoting magical practices associated with personal power.

The serenity prayer mentioned earlier does not have the expectations of an immediate cure or of global improvement. Some things can be changed, some not, and there is a difference that must be perceived. Knowing the difference then may contribute to the process of recovery and it is this discernment on the part of the sufferer that is important.

Prayer, however, is used increasingly in approaches to healing, is related to specific health outcomes (Duckro and Magaletta 1994; McCullough 1995) and is acceptable within medical practice itself (Magaletta and Duckro 1996). Vande-Creek, Rogers and Lester (1999) found both an interest in and practice of prayer as a complementary therapy for breast cancer outpatients.

Dossey (1993) has dedicated a complete book to prayer and advocates its use within clinical medical practice, providing a wealth of critical research support. He also comes to the conclusion that prayer for a specific result rarely works predictably and that the injunction of 'Thy will be done' is the most efficacious of non-directed prayer, citing the work of Bruce Klingbeil in the Spindrift papers (Klingbeil 1993). As Dossey notes, non-directive prayer is for the best state of the individual and that may be death (p.99). No doubt we will soon see prayer books with health warnings! This is essentially the act of submission to a higher power that we found in the last chapter, combined with an intention to be healed. If we couple this to the serenity prayer, then we have a chain of attitudes that includes submission, intention and the knowledge of difference. In perhaps what are now old-fashioned terms, these could be translated as humility, steadfastness and discernment, all personal qualities of being which no doubt have physiological sequelae, but work at a quite different level of experience and consequence.

Prayer in the above sense is something which an individual does for himself, not that another person does for him. This is an important distinction to make. In the various spiritual healing endeavours mentioned below, it is not necessarily the individual who is encouraged to submit his prayers but healers who direct energies, or skilled prayers who pray for the patient, that are involved in the healing. The patient is recipient. In contrast, for the drinker, it is the patient, the sufferer, who is brought to prayer by his fellow former sufferer. But it is the patient who prays. While a higher power or energy is involved, it is very much the act of a petitioner initially who calls for that power. This is not to dismiss the prayers of the other and the context of friendship. They act as container, as the setting for healing, but it is the drinker who prays for help. The patient's submission and loss of self before a higher power is the important factor in the process of healing. The relational context is vital and part of the process, but it is important not to confuse the necessary friend with the essential act. We can see how submission may be problematic in a modern context if the person praying is a woman and the setting is traditional. She is asked to submit before a masculine God, sometimes described as 'Father'. For women who have struggled to escape from under male dominance and established an identity of their own, it is surely psychologically difficult to submit to a male gendered divinity and simultaneously lose a sense of self. This is where new forms of religious expression are positive in that they offer alternative perspectives on a non-gendered or female divinity. Submission, however, remains. This is no simple matter. Culture plays an important role. Black women with cancer, for example, rely on religiousness as a coping resource to a greater extent than white women with cancer (Bourjolly 1998). Therefore traditional church-based religious coping resources will provide a valuable framework of support. Similarly, the elderly sick and depressed use church-based religious resources as an effective coping resource (Koenig, George and Peterson 1998a; Koenig, Pargament and Nielsen 1998b). The expression of spirituality will find its own form according to the person, the cultural setting and the temporal context.

Church settings or religious groups offer the petitioner the chance to behave differently in a community context and for the community to treat that person differently too, as long as the communal system of meanings is supported. Where traditional religious systems and theologies have adopted hierarchies and dogma, there is a current rejection by some in favour of privatized meanings and self-responsibility. The implication for healing is that it too becomes a personal responsibility, but instead of a local community group, where personal acts can be contributed for the benefits of others, the healing becomes privatized and personalized.

A prayer answered

Believers insist that prayers are answered, but those answers are intended to be instrumental for the person praying or those witnessing that prayer, and not evidential for a broader group. Prayers can have a material outcome and may be surprising in this outcome as they work upon the consciousness of the receiver as the following story tells.

A colleague told me of a time when he was convinced that his calling in life was to have a house and a garden to which people would come and be healed. He would simply administer this house and garden. In the house people would learn to meditate, be fed, accommodated and cared for materially and spiritually as in traditional concepts of hospitality and sanctuary. A house would be a place for the weary to lay his head, gain respite from the burdens of life and rest awhile.

In the garden, the visitor could sit and partake of a calm and peaceful life enjoying the simple pleasures and senses of the flowers, the earth and the various creatures. It would be a haven from the world where visitors could retreat and find themselves in relationship to a broader ecology, working with the soil, experiencing the changes of the weather directly on their skin, harvesting directly from the ground: a return to that consciousness of unity by listening to its subtle call. What was grown in the garden could be used in the kitchen of the house; a garden for healing and rejuvenation, reciprocal to the house and a source of higher knowledge and insight. He would be no teacher but a caretaker and gardener.

After several years of trying to convert this dream into reality, of discussing various funding strategies and all of them failing, he decided that, in his best interest, it was time to pray. Not that he had not prayed before. This time he was desperate. Patience had run out. His veneer of religious piety had cracked. So, one Sunday, becoming increasingly frustrated with officialdom, an awareness that his life was going slowly off the rails and having a sincere wish to serve, in a rather romanticized way, he went to his local church. His prayer was simple, direct and confrontational. It was also from the heart. He demanded of his God, in the way that he told it, that there was to be no more messing about with ambiguity and that he wanted a direct answer. This answer had to be material and immediate and it was crucial to his future faith. Not perhaps the most diplomatic of petitions and certainly rejecting all spiritual advice, except for the sincerity. He had spoken from the heart and it was, as he later learned, symptomatic of an existential crisis that he was denying from himself. In a stunning disregard for the common injunction against using prayer as self-seeking, he demanded a house and a garden. Now.

He received an answer to his prayer, as he understood it, and in a material way. The answer was 'Your body is the house and the world is your garden.' Although his prayer was answered, he had also to live with the ramifications of that prayer. All that he had asked was given to him, yet he had also to see that the resources which he had sought had been always there to fulfil his deepest wish. To take his own wish seriously then, he must do things differently. How he did this is another story, but the meaning here is that even when prayers are fully answered, the matter does not stop at the answer. There are consequences to prayers. Answers are not always comfortable resolutions. This is also an example of prayer resulting in a change of consciousness, the element of transcendence that was discussed in Chapter 2.

This change of awareness, as a result of a prayer being answered, and the working out of the consequences of this awareness take time. This has ramifications for spiritual healing when prayer is involved. There may indeed be profound changes taking place as a result of prayer, but the manifestation of those changes in daily life demands time. When we attempt to separate an event that needs healing from the biography of person and then apply a technique like prayer to heal a problem, we are committing a series of mistakes in understanding both the processes of falling sick and becoming healthy and the spiritual journey of the person involved. Falling sick is part of a personal biography and the search for health is an important part of an individual narrative that will influence her future. It will take time to achieve health outcomes and what those outcomes will be is not easy to predict. The person may remain chronically sick yet consider that their life has indeed changed for the better. In addition, the application of prayer is not equivalent to the administration of medication. McCullough (1995) suggests even that prayer's efficacy as a coping resource may not be realized until distress reaches a sufficient level. We saw this in the alcohol research in Chapter 5.

The petitioner has a spiritual biography too. My colleague above had to live with the consequences of his answered prayer. It brought about an existential change that he first experienced as devastating. But in the broader picture of his life it was essential, or so he says.

If we are to understand prayer and its ramifications for healing, we have to develop an understanding of narratives. The consequences of prayer will be seen materially, but the time-span in which they occur will not always be predictable. We also have to understand the state of the person who is praying. Knowing what to look for is one thing, knowing where to look is another and knowing when to look is yet another.

Spiritual healing research in medical settings

Prayer is only one form of healing that is regarded as spiritual. There is a variety of other forms of spiritual healing and these are comprehensively described by Dossey (1993), Benor (1990, 1991, 1992), Solfin (1984) and Wirth (1995; Wirth and Cram 1997; Wirth et al. 1996a; Wirth et al. 1996b). The National Federation of Spiritual Healers in England (NFSH 1999) define spiritual healing as restoring the balance of body, mind and spirit in the recipient with the intention of promoting self-healing, to bring a sense of well-being and peace to the recipient (p.2). A further description concerns itself with finding an inner peaceful core, connecting with a universal source of peace and love that is channelled for the benefit of another. This connection with a universal force is also at the centre of 'therapeutic touch' and belies its connections with ancient systems of healing (Fischer and Johnson 1999).

While the state of mind necessary for healing has been elusive to research, there has been quite extensive research into the physical sequelae of spiritual healing phenomena which has included investigations using controlled trials (Benor 1990). Enzymes and body chemicals in vitro have been studied, as have the effects of healing on cells and lower organisms (including bacteria, fungus and yeasts), human tissue cells in vitro, the motility of simple organisms and plants, on animals and on human problems. While spiritual healing is often dismissed as purely a placebo response, the evidence from studies of lower organisms and cells would indicate that there is direct influence. Even if we introduce the idea of expectancy effects as an influence on experimental data, we are still left with a body of knowledge which begs understanding (Solfin 1984; Wirth 1995).

In fact the explanations of 'placebo response', 'spontaneous regression' and 'expectancy effect' are no less metaphysical as those given for healing pheno-mena. Why would a yeast, for example, want to please a human experimenter? And if spontaneous regression does occur, when does it occur, under what conditions and why is it occurring less often? Burston (1996) argues, albeit regarding psychiatry, that 'if spontaneous remission started to disappear in the late nineteenth century, there must have been something profoundly unhelpful or even unhealthy about the changing hospital environment' (p.242). Dienstfrey (1999b) asks, 'Why is no one following the placebo?' (p.233), given that it is accepted as a major factor influencing drug studies. Similarly, if spontaneous remission does occur and this is seen as an explanation for spiritual healing, then why have we studied it so little? If by expecting results to occur we can influence those results, then surely this is an important tool regarding health-care practices. If these phenomena are relegated to the area of the paranormal, then the terms themselves cannot be used in conventional explanations simply as short cuts to the dismissal of alternative explanations. Furthermore, using the terms as exp-lanatory principles is intellectually lazy. If, as Burston suggests, it is something to do with the settings in which remission occurs, then we should be focusing our endeavours upon those settings. That we choose the organic milieu in modern medicine is acceptable, but this does not mean that we should remove the relational and social, or the spiritual, in the broader aspects of health-care delivery.

General practice

At the level of daily practice some general practitioners have been willing to entertain the idea of spiritual healing and incorporate it into their practice, to use spiritual explanations for some of their patient contact, or as part of their referral network (Brown 1995; Brown and Sheldon 1989; Cohen 1989; Dossey 1993; Pietroni 1986). Cohen (1989) emphasizes the value of touch, time and com-passion which the healer can offer and the benefits of referral. Such practice points out the value of working together as a referral network of practitioners.

King *et al.* (1992) focused on patients who use faith healers and physicians to care for their medical problems to learn how often physicians see patients who are involved in faith healing, and to learn more about physicians' attitudes and experiences with faith healing. A questionnaire was mailed to 1025 family physicians in seven US states. Approximately one half (52%) of the 594 participating physicians were aware of at least one patient in their practice who had had a faith-healing experience. Most physicians came in contact with such patients no more frequently than once a year; 55 per cent agreed and 20 per cent disagreed that reliance on faith healers often leads to serious medical problems. However, 44 per cent thought that physicians and faith healers can work together to cure some patients and 23 per cent believed that faith healers divinely heal some people whom physicians cannot help. Family physicians were divided in their views about faith healing, with a majority expressing scepticism and a sizeable minority favourable towards it. What was also apparent was that physicians know little about what their patients' believe. As we are beginning to become increasingly aware (Dull and Skokan 1995; Irving *et al.* 1998), those beliefs play a significant role in healing and recovery.

Chronic complaints and recalcitrance

In Brown's (1995) study of chronic problems in an English general practice of six doctors, adult patients with chronic complaints were referred by their GP to a healing clinic. In choosing the patients, the GP included those who had had a problem of six months duration and had not responded well to usual inter- ventions, other secondary referrals or counselling. In my cycle of distress management, such patients would be at Phase III in the escalation of distress (see Figure 6.1). Treatment sessions lasted 20 minutes once a week for an eight week period. The spiritual healing used a 'laying on of hands approach' to 'channel healing energies' and was assessed using a validated quality of life questionnaire that has established population norms for comparison (SF–36). There were significant changes after eight weeks in what was a group of patients with poor health status in role limitations, social function, pain, general health and vitality. These improvements were not extended to an assessment after 26 weeks from the beginning of the study. As the author says, we cannot make any specific conclusions regarding the healing approach as there were no treatment controls. However, for a group of chronic patients, recalcitrant to previous intervention, there was improvement.

In my book regarding suicide, it is this smallest of possible changes that begins a cascade of recovery (see Figure 6.1), if nothing more than promoting the hope that something, however small, is possible. Indeed, rather than expecting massive heroic changes, maybe we would be better educating ourselves and our patients for the smallest possible positive change that could be expected (Aldridge 1988; Aldridge and Rossiter 1983, 1984, 1985; Dallos and Aldridge 1986). A series of small improvements over time is clinically valuable as Brown's study suggests and

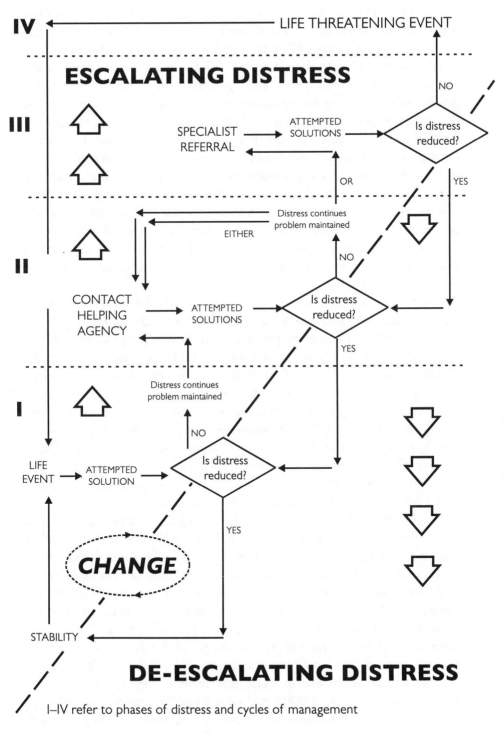

Figure 6.1 Cycles of escalating and de-escalating distress

relevant to the important primary care context of general practice. To recognize a pattern of improvement we would need time-based studies with multiple variables in general practice (Aldridge 1992; Aldridge and Pietroni 1987).

Chronic symptoms in general practice are also the focus of Dixon's study (1998). Like the above study with several general practitioners working together, patients with a condition that had lasted for six months which was unresponsive to treatment were referred to a healer. They were assessed at the beginning of the study, after three months and after six months using the Hospital Anxiety and Depression Scale (Zigmond and Snaith 1983) and the Nottingham Health Profile (Hunt 1985). Anxiety and depression relief is an important general factor in primary health care indicating an improvement in health care (Eisenberg 1992) as it is in general psychiatry (Frances and Borg 1993). Both are implied in the escalation of distress that leads to mood disorder implicated with suicidal behaviour (Lepine *et al.* 1993; Rudd, Dahm and Rajab 1993). A reduction in anxiety and depression may be the initial stages in relieving distress and promoting recovery.

The patients were told that they were going to see a healer rather than a faith or spiritual healer, who would then pass her hands close to the patient, visualizing the passage of light through the patient accompanied by relaxing music. We are not told of the control condition and the use of relaxing music confounds the treatment, given that the use of music as music therapy is a known anxiolytic (Aldridge 1996). However, compared to the control scores, there was an improvement in anxiety and depression scores after three months that was maintained at six months for the treatment group. Functional improvements on the Nottingham Health Profile at three months were not maintained at a significant level after six months. These patients were previously unresponsive to treatment and the improvement in general mood state scores indicates a general setting for recovery that is of worth for clinical practice.

Natural killer cells, as measure of immunological functioning, were also measured in the search for an objective indicator, rather like the Holy Grail of medicine's Avalon. No significant immunological responses were found. This is disappointing for the researchers as the immune response associated with poor mood state is said to be implicated in the cascade of deteriorating health (Dillon and Baker 1985). There is a considerable literature relating immune function to stress and mood disorder (Kiecolt-Glaser *et al.* 1992; Kiecolt-Glaser and Glaser 1988; Solomon 1987; Stein, Keller and Schleifer 1985) and depression and stress as a co-factor in health hazard identification (Kiecolt-Glaser and Glaser 1999).

Pennebaker's study of disclosure and immune function (Pennebaker, Kiecolt-Glaser and Glaser 1988) would suggest that the vital expressive element that the patient performs is missing from this study. If, as mentioned earlier, health is a performed activity, then a change in mood state is a small step forward, but perhaps to see this realized as a change in immune function there needs to be activity on the part of the patient. Immune function must be performed; not just stimulated in the organism, but maintained actively by the organism. That which makes the spiritual 'spiritual' is a transcendence of the current situation through change in meaning, the achievement of consciousness. There may be concomitant changes in health status and these would be expected even at the immune level, but it is a change in understanding and the consequent acts that must surely be taken as evidence for healing. These changes must be achieved and performed by the patient.

A study that may have some relevance here was conducted by a team from the Maharishi University of Management in Iowa, USA (Hagelin *et al.* 1999). They gathered together 4000 participants in the Transcendental Meditation Program in Washington, DC, prospectively to reduce stress and increase coherence in the collective consciousness of the district. The evidence of this reduced stress was to be a fall in homicide, rape and assault crimes during the project. They considered the effects of known confounding variables like the weather, daylight, historical crime trends, annual patterns of crime, crime trends from neighbouring cities and police staffing. Time series analysis showed a peak drop in assault crimes by 23 per cent controlling for temperature and allowing for a regression to mean. As the group of meditators increased in size during the eight-week period (the group began with less than a thousand, reached 2500 members at week 5 and 4000 by week 7), the assault crime rate dropped progressively.

There was no contact between the members of the group and the general population. Yet, if there is an influence upon community coherence which results in reduction in stress, then this would indicate the appropriate level at which such interventions should be made; not individuals but populations.

These studies mark for me what is a continuing problem with the use of so-called spiritual healing. The patient is always passive. Energies are channelled by the healer. Intercessory prayers intercede on behalf of the patient. Meditators influence consciousness. Yet we saw in the previous chapters that it is the involvement of the patient that is necessary in performing health. Prayer as a spiritual activity is undertaken by the patient herself, not something that must necessarily be applied to her. Until this is recognized then the logical corollary is that we assess the healers and the prayers, not the patients, for change. If prayer is efficacious, then surely those praying or partaking of energy are benefiting too and it is here that we would expect to see change. It would make as much sense to measure the healers and meditators as it does the recipients.

A broader ecology of care

The demand for whole person treatment has been strenuously adopted by some nursing groups who remind us that in caring for the patient there is a need to include spiritual needs and to allow their expression (Boutell and Bozett 1990; Burkhardt 1989; Clark and Dawson 1996; Dossey 1999; Ferrell et al. 1998; Grasser and Craft 1984; Harrington, Lackey and Gates 1996; Labun 1988; Magaletta and Duckro 1996; Potts 1996; Rukholm et al. 1991; Rustoen and Hanestad 1998; Soeken and Carson 1987). Within these approaches there is a core of opinion which accepts that suffering and pain are part of a larger life experience, and that they can have meaning for the patient and for the carer(s) (Nagai Jacobson and Burkhardt 1989). The emphasis is placed upon the person's concept of God, sources of strength and hope, the significance of religious practices and rituals for the patient and their belief system (Soeken and Carson 1987). As we read earlier, prayer is a form of expression and allows the utterance of a broad spectrum of needs.

When the goal of treatment is palliative, in terminally ill cancer patients with a prognosis of six months or less, the most important outcome is improving patient quality of life (Greisinger et al. 1997). Interviews with 120 terminally ill cancer patients showed that their most important concerns encompass existential, spiritual, familial, physical and emotional issues and that throughout their illness these concerns were rarely a focus of their care. What is of further concern is that doctors underestimate symptom severity 15 per cent of the time (Stephens et al. 1997). This has important implications for palliative interventions and the way in which patient understandings are taken seriously.

Doctors, nurses and clergy have worked together to care for the dying (Conrad 1985; Greisinger et al. 1997; McMillan and Weitzner 1998; Reed 1987; Roche 1989) and a community team approach which includes the family of the patient and his or her friends appears to be beneficial (Aldridge 1987a, 1987b, 1987c, 1987d) (see Table 6.3). These principle benefits are concerned with a lessening of state–trait anxiety, general feelings of well-being and an increasing spiritual awareness for the dying person regardless of gender, marital status, age or diagnosis (Kaczorowski 1989). This does not imply that each practitioner has to address all of these components, rather that those involved identify what is necessary for the patient and can call upon the appropriate resources. The nurse specializing in pain management works with the priest understanding suffering and together with the patient who is in pain. But the patient plays an active contributory role. Technical support is vital, but optimal care involves emotional support, which may include techniques of relaxation, visualization and meditation (Peteet et al. 1992).

Table 6.3 Family change and terminal illness	
Coping with physical changes	Anticipation of pain Management of pain Management of the physical sequelae of illness (nausea, incontinence) and change in physical appearance Management of the physical sequelae of treatment
Coping with personal changes	Loss of hope, fitness and identity Anxiety and depression about the future Loss of role in family and in employment Frustration and helplessness
Coping with family and marital changes	Resolution of conflict Change in parental roles Anxiety about the future welfare (emotional and financial) Anticipated hospital contacts and treatment Anticipated loss of a family member Planning the future Social isolation Changes in family boundary, and of family and marital emotional distance Negotiation of dependence/independence Saying 'goodbye' and talking about dying Handling the above personal and physical changes Loss of sexual activity
Coping with spiritual changes	Feelings of loss, alienation and abandonment Understanding suffering Accepting dependency Handling anger and frustration Forgiving others Discovering peace Discussing death Grieving Planning the funeral Discovering the value of living

It must be emphasized that these changes have ramifications through the interconnected systems. Personal changes have implications for family and community members.

A team perspective also allows us to care for the caregivers. In working with the dying it becomes clear that in the long term we need to look after those people involved in the team itself (Aldridge 1987d; Thomas 1989). Stressors and health risks in the medical profession are well documented but seldom openly discussed (Sonneck and Wagner 1996). Very often a 'conspiracy of silence' about these stressors exists which is allowed to continue because of denial and defensiveness. The most important stressors in the medical system result from the treatment of and care for patients. Other stressors are team conflicts, insecurity, lack of autonomy, large workload and increasing criticisms, expectations and demands from the public. In addition, female doctors complain about the strain they experience in emergency services. They also suffer especially from the role strain between job stressors and family responsibilities. Signs of these double stressors can already be seen early in the medical course and mark the whole career of female doctors. Compared to the general population, the overall mortality rate of doctors decreased during the last decade, but is still worse than that of other professionals of comparable education. In particular the suicide rates are high, for males two to three times that of the general population, for females as much as five to six times. There is a high proportion of psychiatric diseases, particularly addiction and depression, among doctors. As Sonneck and Wagner (1996) write, 'We must keep in mind, that, despite being "gods in white", a medical degree does not infer immunity to mental illness, drug addiction, alcoholism, or other self-destructive behaviors' (p.255).

Jean and the men in her life

Jean had a massive tumour on her spine that had spread to her lungs. She used a variety of methods for pain relief including pharmacological and psychological. She also tried meditation and her priest came to pray. Her general practitioner was interested in such forms of communal intervention and visited when the sacraments of the Christian eucharist were being administered or when there was a session of meditation and guided imagery. So did her immediate family, at first. Then her parents just happened to be there. Sometimes neighbours would, by chance, drop in to visit.

Jean's situation deteriorated. She wished to remain at home, however. Friends were calling regularly to her house and she found the situation enlivening rather than tiring, which was unusual. One day, her husband, her priest and her general practitioner were concerned that she was not talking about death. Given that a priority of spiritual counselling was acknowledging death and coming to terms with it, all three thought that something was going wrong. Jean was in denial, as they saw it, and for things to move on maybe someone should talk to her about it.

When Jean was gently asked if she wanted to talk about dying, she said 'No.' Dying for her was self-evident. She had to live with it all the time, but she was sure that her husband, her priest and her general practitioner needed to talk about it and could they be counselled as she could no longer protect them from the inevitable. Given what we know about burnout and stress among healing professionals, particularly doctors, Jean's insight is valuable. How do we care for those in the caring professions?

Jean died; a poor health-care outcome. Her sons, husband and family mourned and recovered. They remembered the sessions when people visited, how people struggled not to sneeze during meditations and how they were crammed in, sitting on the stairs. The general practitioner lost a patient, but he was surprised how little she suffered and was pleased that her immediate family were doing so well. The quality of her life as she was dying was the best we could provide. Perhaps a good outcome after all? Certainly not easily measurable. We can count one death. But the relief of suffering, the ability to go on for the family, the absence of problems, how do we assess these? Yet any practitioner will recognize what is being said.

While such a grouping of practitioners and friends may have no immediate financial validity, we need to ask whether there are perhaps community priorities that have an experiential validity that is also valid and necessary. The problem is that if we cannot assess such an element then we are unlikely to meet the patient's need for it (Higginson, Wade and McCarthy 1992). Perhaps it is easier for patients to understand death than it is for health-care experts to understand transcendence.

Increasing numbers of patients with cancer are being cared for by home caregivers (Hileman, Lackey and Hassanein 1992). The primary purpose of Hileman's study was to identify, categorize and assess the importance of needs expressed by 492 home caregivers and to determine how well they were satisfied. Caregivers, unpaid people who helped with physical care or coping with the disease process, were selected from the records of two non-profit community cancer agencies and two hospital outpatient oncology clinics. Six need categories were identified: psychological, informational, patient care, personal, spiritual and household. Those needs changed over time and required frequent reassessment, but it was the caregivers as well as the patients who were seen as in need. If we continually refine our outcome measures to assess the individual patient then we are committing a big mistake by ignoring his ecological milieu.

With an increasing number of women surviving breast cancer beyond treatment, the focus of care has shifted from the acute treatment related side effects to long-term effects associated with changes in quality of life (Ferrell et al. 1998). Improving or maintaining the quality of life for persons with cancer is a major goal of end-of-life care (McMillan and Weitzner 1998). Data collected from home care hospice patients with cancer (n = 255) and a group of apparently healthy adults in the community (n = 32) confirmed three categories of need: psychophysiological, functional and social/spiritual well-being. Patients are able to appraise their functional abilities realistically and still maintain their social network and spiritual beliefs. Indeed, patients give family relationships and spiritual beliefs greater focus during a terminal illness.

Providing information, emotional support, behavioural training in coping skills, psychotherapy (of various kinds), and, more speculatively, spiritual/existential therapy are prioritized in increasing importance by Cunningham and Edmonds (1996).

In a three-month study of the perceived needs and anxiety levels of 166 adult family members of intensive care unit (ICU) patients (Rukholm *et al.* 1991), family needs and situational anxiety were significantly related. Worries, trait anxiety, age and family needs explained 38 per cent of the variation of situational anxiety. In addition, spiritual needs and situational anxiety explained 33 per cent of the variation of family needs. In threatening situations, families need strategies to cope. As Zigmond (1987) writes: 'On our own, or in our most intimate groups, we devise more personal and idiosyncratic beliefs, rituals and protocols to ward off the potential storms or deserts of uncertainty' (p.69). The spiritual dimension, while perhaps not warding off uncertainty, offers a satisfactory strategy by which uncertainty may be understood and coped with. This would surely be transcendence.

Ambiguity in outcomes

Richards and Folkman (1997) found spiritual phenomena were spontaneously reported in interviews of 68 of 125 recently bereaved HIV positive and HIV negative partners of men who died from AIDS. Spiritual understandings helped assimilate the fact of death and were appraised as sources of solace and meaning. Those reporting spiritual phenomena also showed higher levels of depression and anxiety and lower levels of positive states of mind, used more adaptive coping strategies and reported more physical health symptoms than those who did not report spiritual phenomena. While these findings are with partners of patients, it reflects the work of King, Speck and Thomas (1999), who found that stronger spiritual belief is an independent predictor of poor outcome at nine months for patients admitted to the acute services of a London hospital. Chronic pain patients who endorse a greater use of prayer to cope with their pain also reported a greater degree of disability (Ashby and Lenhart 1994). While the causal relations between use of prayer and outcomes or disability cannot be adequately understood, we might well be advised to heed this warning that associations with spirituality are not always benign and there are ambiguities to be explained.

There is a story told of a religious man who lost in spiritual reverie – some might call this unawareness of pragmatic reality – falls off a sea cliff. On his way down he grabs at a branch and, as fortune will have it, he breaks his fall. Clinging to the branch, hanging precipitously from the cliff, he prays for help. Confirmed in the belief that sincere prayer will save him, his prayers increase in intensity. At that moment a boat appears and the crew hail him to let go and they will pick him from the waters below. 'No thank you,' he replies, 'I am a religious man and God will save me.' The crew plead with him, but eventually respecting his right of religious freedom, they go on their way.

The man prays harder, using all the names of the divine that he can remember and every esoteric invocation that he has previously studied. Being a scholar of such matters and given that his plight was brought about by a state of religious reverie, he knows that help will come. He trusts that knowledge gleaned in a lifetime of study. At that moment, the coastguard helicopter appears intent on rescue. He waves them away furiously. 'No thank you,' he says, 'My spiritual beliefs are such that God will save me. I trust in his promise.' His would-be rescuers, having no mandate to intervene against his beliefs and wishes and not wanting to come between a man and his maker, leave.

Eventually, his strength fails, partly exacerbated by vigorously waving help away and vehemently protesting his beliefs. He falls to the sea below and dies. On entering heaven, he asks why his prayer was not answered and why God did not rescue him. The reply was that his prayer was answered twice; first a boat was sent and then a helicopter.

The danger of promoting understandings and calling them spiritual is that they may deflect from the really pragmatic understandings which are necessary for daily life. An essential element of spiritual understanding is discernment of applicability, not the repetition of vain exercises and wishful thinking. The impulse behind the development of modern analgesics may be as divine as the exercise of meditative techniques, as Jean found. Knowing when and how to use them is the important factor.

In the same vein of argument, there is concern that some patients are being promised fantastic healings by spiritual healers and are also being told that they are not recovering either because they do not want to or that they do not love others enough, or that they are secretly resisting the healer. Such approaches are simply wrong, as is the advice to refrain from conventional medicine. As in the preceding anecdote, conventional medicine may be the boat that is sent to help as an answer to prayer. It does not mean that other options are to be discarded. Discernment is the key. For those seeking miracles or some sort of magical intervention and the exposition of healing powers, this approach is disappointing. It involves no dressing up in special clothes, nor any fancy hand passes or magical incantations. Indeed transvestism, dressing up in clothes inappropriate to the period or the local culture, is a warning of spiritual bankruptcy, not enhanced powers (Marsham 1990), as is the use of languages strange to the culture.

Spirituality in the treatment of persons living with AIDS

Comprehensive treatment programmes for people living with AIDS recommend that the spiritual welfare of the patient, and its influence on their well-being, is included (Belcher, Dettmore and Holzemer 1989; Flaskerud and Rush 1989; Gutterman 1990; Hall 1998; Holt *et al.* 1999; Kaplan, Marks and Mertens 1997; Ribble 1989; Sowell and Misener 1997; Warner-Robbins and Christiana 1989).

Individuals who were spiritually well and able to find meaning and purpose in their lives were also found to be hardier (Carson and Green 1992). In taking an ecological perspective that considers the sufferer and the caregivers, Cooke (1992) reminds us that the care of HIV-infected patients is demanding and the emotional consequences of caring for HIV-infected people should be directly addressed. We have then a variety of needs to meet and, as we saw in Chapter 5, the emphasis on spiritual welfare is not simply on the patient but also includes the caregiver. Other authors, while supporting an emphasis on the spiritual, also direct our attention to the confounding problem of religions that condemn sexual activity and the ramifications this has for the person living with HIV or AIDS (Jenkins 1995).

While the term spiritual healing is used here within the context of orthodox medical practices as a complementary or adjuvant approach and as an additional factor for inclusion, the term spirit has other applications. In the absence of a medical cure for AIDS, HIV-infected individuals may seek alternative treatments and folk healing practices. In inner city New Jersey, HIV-infected Hispanics, aged 23 to 55, receiving care at an HIV/AIDS clinic, and primarily of Puerto Rican origin or descent, believed in good and evil spirits and that such spirits had a causal role in their infection, either alone or in conjunction with the AIDS virus (Suarez, Raffaelli and OLeary 1996). They sought spiritual folk healing for physical relief, spiritual relief and protection from evil. A minority hoped for cure. We must be aware of the prevalence of folk beliefs and alternative healing practices and cannot assume when we talk of spiritual healing that it will fit into the sanitized views of a rationalized Western approach.

The elderly

Prayer is described by several authors as valuable in terms of care for the elderly across several cultures (Chatters and Taylor 1989; Foley, Wagner and Waskel 1998; Garrett 1991; Gorham 1989; Koenig et al. 1989, 1997; Markides 1983; Reed 1987; Taylor and Chatters 1991).

The seeking of medical help and prayer are not mutually exclusive (Bearon and Koenig 1990), as prayer is considered to be an active coping response in the face of stressful medical problems. A study of 160 physicians found that physicians believe religion has a positive effect on physical health, that religious issues should be addressed and that the older patient may ask the physician to pray with them (Koenig et al. 1989). An influential factor in this questioning is the belief system of the practitioner, which may influence in turn the willingness of the patient to talk about such matters.

As we saw in the cancer research earlier, spiritual factors are important for the caregivers. The study by Chang et al. (1998) examines how religious and spiritual coping is related to specific conditions of caregiving and psychological distress among informal caregivers to community-residing disabled elders. Spiritual coping strategies influence caregiver distress indirectly through the quality of the relationship between caregiver and care recipient. Caregivers who used religious or spiritual beliefs to cope with caregiving had a better relationship with those who were being cared for, which is associated with lower levels of depression and an increased dedication to the role of caring.

Hope

In a recent paper assessing the motivation of oncology patients concerning their use of complementary therapies, patients reported psychological benefits such as hope and optimism (Downer *et al.* 1994). The authors conclude that hope is an important issue which fosters a more collaborative approach to management. While being a word in common parlance, the term 'hope' is not commonly voiced in the world of medicine. However, palliative care has a tradition of breadth in its understanding of health-care needs and we find throughout the literature that the spiritual needs of patients are mentioned, with hope often in the foreground.

We know from clinical practice that the will to live is an important factor. Purpose and meaning in life are vital and all too often are not questioned when we are in good health. But should we fall ill, then purpose and meaning become crucial to survival. Illness may be seen as a step on life's way that brings us in contact with who we really are. The positive aspect of suffering has been neglected in our modern scientific culture such that we, as practitioners and patients, often search for immediate relief. While the management of cancer pain has been a major contribution of the hospice movement, the understanding of suffering is still elusive in the literature. It may well be that the difficulties reported in effectively relieving pain are the result of the failure to identify suffering.

We are all asked the ultimate question of what meaning and purpose our lives would have had if we were to die now. Most of our activities cut us off from this brutal confrontation, or are an attempt to shield us from this realization. While the management of pain is often a scientific and technical task, the relief of suffering is an existential task. In the major spiritual traditions suffering has always had the potential to transform the individual. As Tournier (Dawson 1997) reminds us, it is love that has the power to change the sign of suffering from negative to positive.

Maintaining integrity and hope

Positive emotions, which include the qualitative aspects of life – hope, joy, beauty and unconditional love – are known to be beneficial for the process of coping, both with a challenging diagnosis, during the course of treatment and for post-operative recovery.

A significant beneficial factor in enhancing the quality of life is hope. Hope has been identified as a multifaceted phenomenon that is a valuable human response, even in the face of a severe reduction in life expectation. Yates (Davis and Robinson 1996) offers six dimensions of hope: the sensations and emotions of expectancy and confidence; a cognitive dimension that comprises positive perceptions and a belief that a desired outcome is realistically possible; a behavioural dimension where patients act on their positive beliefs to achieve their desires; a contextual dimension that links expectations with those of the family and friends; and a temporal dimension looking forwards or even backwards.

Hope is defined by the nurse-researcher Herth (Estes 1991; Hay and Morisy 1985) as an 'inner power directed toward enrichment of "being"'. In her study of hope in the dying, with the exception of those diagnosed with AIDS, overall hope levels among subjects were high and found to remain stable over time. Seven hope-fostering categories (interpersonal connectedness, attainable aims, spiritual base, personal attributes, light-heartedness, uplifting memories and affirmation of worth) and three hope-hindering categories (abandonment and isolation, uncontrollable pain and discomfort, devaluation of personhood) were identified.

Hope, like prayer (Crombez and Dubreuco 1991), is a coping strategy used by those confronted with a chronic illness that involves an expectation going beyond visible facts and seen as a motivating force to achieve inner goals. These goals change. While a distant future of life expectancy no longer exists for AIDS patients, life aims can be redefined and refocused. With the progression of physical deterioration then the future becomes less defined in terms of the body and time, but in the meaning attached to life events in relationship with family and friends. In later stages there is a shift towards less concrete goals and a refocusing on the self to include the inner peace and serenity necessary for dying (Hay and Morisy 1985).

The true meaning of hope is that of an inclination towards something which we do not know. There is a longing for the unknown. We are all waiting for a change – even if it is a material change of circumstance – and this expectation is hope. Such hope cannot be touched and often cannot be understood. It is an attainment that may be described as beyond happiness and above death.

Any therapeutic tasks must concentrate on the restoration of hope, accommodating feelings of loss, isolation and abandonment, understanding suffering, forgiving others, accepting dependency while remaining independent and making sense of dying. Hope, when submitted to the scrutiny of the psychologist and not conforming to an established reality, can easily be interpreted as denial. For the therapist, hope is a replacement for therapeutic nihilism enabling us to offer constructive effort and sound expectations (Burns 1991).

Prayer in medicine

Although initial clinical research into the benefits of prayer was inconclusive (Collipp 1969; Joyce and Welldon 1965; Rosner 1975) more recent studies, from a broader medical perspective and with larger study populations, have shown that intercessory prayer is beneficial. Several authors argue that religious variables are relevant, even if not beneficial, and that physicians should choose to attend to them (Dossey 1993; King and Dein 1998; King 1997; King et al. 1999; Magaletta and Duckro 1996).

In a study by Saudia et al. (1991), the relationship between health locus of control and helpfulness of prayer as a direct-action coping mechanism in patients before having cardiac surgery was examined. The Multidimensional Health Locus of Control Scales and the investigator developed Helpfulness of Prayer Scale were issued to 100 subjects on the day before cardiac surgery. Ninety-six subjects indicated that prayer was used as a coping mechanism in dealing with the stress of cardiac surgery and 70 of these subjects gave it the highest possible rating on the Helpfulness of Prayer Scale. Prayer was perceived as a helpful, direct-action coping mechanism and was independent of whether individuals believed that their lives were controlled by themselves or a powerful other. The importance of this study is that it emphasizes prayer as direct action that the individual uses as a coping strategy.

In a coronary care unit the prayer group had an overall better outcome requiring less antibiotics, diuretics and intubation/ventilation than control (Byrd 1988). For renal patients, prayer and looking at the problem objectively were used most in coping with stress (Sutton and Murphy 1989). It is interesting to see that at the pragmatic level of the patient, prayer and looking at the problem objectively are not exclusive but complementary activities in a system of beliefs. This is not stress reduction correlated with immunological parameters but stress relief as a coping strategy correlated with cognitive factors.

In the treatment of alcoholism there has been an historical influence of spiritual considerations being included in treatment plans (Bergmark 1998; Carroll 1993; Eisenbach-Stagl 1998; McCarthy 1984) apart from the temperance movement. Such treatments for alcohol abuse were often composite packages using physical methods of relaxation, psychological methods of suggestion and auto-suggestion, social methods of group support and service to the community and spiritual techniques of prayer. Such procedures are still in use today and have been extended into the realm of chemical dependency and substance abuse (Buxton, Smith and Seymour 1987; Green, Fullilove and Fullilove 1998; Mathew et al. 1996; Miller 1998b; Navarro et al. 1997; Peteet 1993). Individuals suffering from substance problems are found to have a low level of religious involvement, and spiritual engagement appears to be correlated with recovery (Miller 1998b) while religiosity may be an advantageous coping factor (Kendler, Gardner and Prescott 1997).

Byrd's study

Randolph Byrd's study (1988) at the San Francisco General Hospital has achieved landmark status in the topography of healing research. He asked whether intercessory prayer to a Judeo-Christian God has an effect on the patient's recovery and medical condition while in hospital and, if there is an effect, what are its characteristics. The hypothesis is that intercessory prayer mediates the process of healing. Some might want to add 'if you choose the right god' to this hypothesis, given Byrd's 'born again Christian' approach.

Intercessory prayer was taken as the treatment method for the 192 randomly allocated patients; another 201 patients formed a control group. All 393 patients had standard medical care as expected. The intercessors were 'born again' Christians with an active Christian life of daily devotional prayer who partook of fellowship in their local churches. Each patient was randomized to between three to seven intercessors who were given the patient's first name, diagnosis and general condition. The prayer was done from outside the hospital and is prayer at a distance. Each intercessor was asked to pray daily for a rapid recovery and for the prevention of complications and death. Physicians were informed of the trial but did not know to which group the patients belonged.

Standard medical treatment was given throughout. This is an important point to state as some religious groups see prayer as spiritual healing and medical science as oppositional. Recourse to medical treatment is seen as a weakness in faith and therefore undermining healing, as we will see later in the chapter.

At first glance the statistical results of Byrd's study are impressive with an overall improvement being attributed to prayer. It does indeed show a touching faith on the behalf of medical scientists in statistical results, partly because the results make medical sense. There is less congestive heart failure, cardio-pulmonary arrest and pneumonia, fewer antibiotics are needed, less diuretic medication and less ventilator support. If statistical significance of results were the only criteria then psi phenomena would be widely accepted (Inglis 1979) and healing energies would be incorporated into a conventional approach (Benor 1992).

Looking deeper at these results, anomalies begin to appear. As we have seen earlier, prayer is not an homogeneous practice, nor is it exclusive. As Byrd says in the study itself (p.826) some of the patients in the control group would be prayed for. What we do not know, and this related to my earlier point about prayer and its efficacy for the sufferer, is how many of these patients were praying for themselves and what they were praying for. We know from other studies that many people do pray when sick, and not all of them to a Judeo-Christian God. So it would make sense to know what the prayer activities of the patients were in both treatment and control groups. Furthermore, besides not knowing what the optimal dose-response relationship for prayer is, we do not know at what stage on the spiritual journey were these sufferers and intercessors. When medical circumstances become dire, spiritual needs come to the fore, as we have seen, but these can be indicative of a poorer outcome (King *et al.* 1999).

These intercessory prayers were also made at a distance, the intercessor being absent from the location of the patient. Dossey (1982) has written about the challenge of space time concepts for medicine and particularly in terms of understanding prayer (Dossey 1993). What is important here is that while distant healing is part of a long spiritual tradition, it is also seen as a highly developed form of spiritual healing. Khan (1974), writing about spiritual healing, mentions healing by charms, the use of magnetized water, healing by breathing, healing by magnetized passes, healing by touch, healing by glance, healing by suggestion, healing by presence, healing by prayer and absent healing. The ability to perform absent healing, or healing at a distance, is only possible after the healer has practised healing for a certain time successfully. It is an advanced ability in a sequence of attainments. Yet, we do not know if the intercessors in the Byrd study were chosen for their abilities to heal based on previous practice, extensive experience or that they had the gift of healing.

That this healing took place at a distance effectively rules out that necessary relational context we saw earlier. These Christian did not know the people they were praying for except by first names. To do this study justice in assessing the effect of intercessory prayer Byrd would have needed to study the people doing the praying.

Other authors question why only 6 out of the possible 26 variables showed improvement (Duckro and Magaletta 1994; McCullough 1995). They ask if the improvement were the result of a subgroup within the treatment cohort or was this a result of a general modest improvement (McCullough 1995). We are not told if having seven intercessors is better than having three. Similarly, the specific variables to be prayed for are not given to the intercessors. Rapid recovery was prayed for and Dossey (1993) points out that there was no difference between the two groups on this variable.

Like previous prayer studies, I fear we are demanding such a limited cause–effect relationship that these studies are really controlled trials of wishful thinking rather than the effects of prayer as a spiritual healing. By restricting variables and ignoring the time dimension, misperceiving spiritual development in both healer and patient, then we are simply demonstrating a lack of knowledge of the healing process and the true value of prayer.

The Spindrift papers

The Spindrift papers (Klingbeil 1993) are also used as a series of landmark experiments in spiritual healing research. They graphically illustrate the difficulty faced in presenting an alternative view of reality. The authors were Christian Science practitioners determined to convince the world that the power of prayer, or in their terms 'holy thought', is essential for healing, although they fall out with the rest of the Christian Science Church to which they belonged. Seventeen of the twenty-four collected papers in volume one are written by the Klingbeil father and son team.

When the foreword of a book begins, 'Out of the sordid political fighting of a slowly dying church have come what may be experimental links between the probabilistic nature of quantum mechanics and the prayer healing practices of many devout Christians', then it is safe to assume that the reader is not likely to be assailed by a neutral text concerned with presenting a balanced scientific argument to which we are accustomed. Indeed, many of the chapters repeat the story of the demise of Bruce Klingbeil who, setting out to test the effect of prayer on yeasts and plants experimentally, was subsequently forbidden to carry out the work and then expelled from the Church. Spindrift, and its supporters in other religious movements, have apparently consequently suffered penalties from their respective churches for their views. This complaint appears in paper after paper of the Spindrift collection and, through repetition, rather than eliciting support for the researchers, provokes a counter-reaction. Constantly repeating that they are hard done by, for what the authors see as pioneering work in a scientific field which will have vast implications for clinical medicine, is annoying and detracts from any worthwhile initiatives that may be present in their research.

The main feature of the work is a series of experiments which demonstrate the power of prayer to influence the growth rate of seedlings under stress, the production of carbon dioxide in yeasts and the effect of conscious and unconscious thought on physical systems, reflecting the vast range of experimental work done in parapsychology (Inglis 1979; Solfin 1984). The authors conclude that there is an unconscious counter-force which obscures the positive healing power of prayer, thereby explaining the difficulties of replicating various previous healing endeavours. This negative force is called 'a defence mechanism' and described as evil.

What is of value in their work is the insistence that rather than measuring seedling growth as such, they measure the effect of prayer on the seedlings as they return to normal growth under challenge. Such an observation fits modern ecological thinking.

This research serves as a perfect example of the difficulties facing the consideration of alternative realities, particularly when the researchers seek to justify themselves as valid in a context other than their own. Even within their own original reference group, the authors were ostracized because experimental justification of a 'scientific' claim was regarded as heretical.

There are numerous groups of individuals involved in alternative healing enterprises who feel just as badly handled by what they perceive to be the established orthodoxies of religion, science and medicine. Railing against injustice may help in the short term, but when such woe is expressed as a litany of rejections then even ears sympathetic to their cause may close. Most scientific researchers who do get published have suffered a series of rebuffs, rebuttals and severe intellectual maulings at the hands of journal editors and their peers. Fortunately this is what strengthens the value of the work when it is eventually published. Presenting the work for validation by a larger public in a journal necessarily demands that there will be some challenges to the personal ego of the writer. His or her deeply cherished ideas are likely to be critically questioned. In a liberal culture, where there is a variety of publishing possibilities, such rigorous questioning is healthy. Challenge, when not debilitating, ensures that sound work appears in the foreground and the ego of the author is relegated to the background. Most of us write with a passionate belief in what we are doing. Usually we are held in check from inflicting the excesses of those beliefs on others by the exercise of editorial restraint and peer review. To reject the criticism of peers is either an heroic self-belief in an eternal truth hidden from the rest of the world or simple vanity. Sadly Klingbeil and his son committed suicide, so strong was their feeling of rejection.

A major failing of this work is that some of the papers, in their bitterness and stridency, undermine the very basic tenets of what the authors preach; that is, in Christian Science, thought is all and shapes the physical world (Baker Eddy 1971/1875). Paradoxically, the style in which the Spindrift papers is presented seriously impedes the acceptance of the experimental work which the authors have so laboriously performed. Their thoughts negate their work. Indeed, perhaps the tenets of their work are upheld in the end in that their negative thoughts destroyed the authors.

Frohock (1993) gives a very apt example of a Christian Science couple who, despairing for their sick child who is being conventionally treated in hospital, realize that their thinking is wrong and that the child is indeed made perfect. At this realization, they visit the child in hospital to find that he has dramatically recovered, to the astonishment of the attending physician. Maybe such a realization by the Spindrift authors would have helped in the acceptance of their material efforts and perhaps have saved their own lives.

Miracles and healing

Mary Baker Eddy founded the Christian Science Church over a century ago, arguing that only mind is real and that each person should be her own physician. All faith must be put in the power of prayer to heal and in trusting matter, we distrust spirit, emphasizing the rift between mind and body (May 1995). A similar situation occurs in other fundamentalist movements where miraculous healing is emphasized. Every moment of existence is thought to be the opportunity for a miracle to occur, and through miracles non-believers will be converted to the faith (Smolin 1995). Sickness, from such a perspective, is caused through having a wrong or sinful attitude. We have seen earlier in Chapter 5 that this understanding actually alienates people from the divine. There is no cosmic law of cause and effect regarding sin and sickness. Christian Science, in calling itself a 'science', may try to invoke the impression that such laws are known, yet simultaneously refuses to submit itself, as a science, to such proof.

We know that many people who are sick pray and consult a practitioner. Their practitioners may refer them to a spiritual healer or a secondary source of healing. Condemning them as sinners is not only an inappropriate theology but plainly unbiblical. The ineffective prayer of the righteous regarding healing is the common experience; not because the prayers are weak or the petitioner is a sinner (given that from a Christian perspective we are all sinners). Prophets, saints and spiritual masters have all accepted lives with a physical ailment. Indeed, the recognized spiritual masters from a variety of traditions in the twentieth century have died of diseases like heart failure and cancer (Dossey 1993; Parker 1997).

While the dying may gain peace through prayer, eradicating disease through such petitions has not happened. Job, in the Christian Bible, loses all his belongings, his family and his health although being a faithful believer. Eventually, after fruitless advice from his friends and counsellors, in a dialogue with his God, he admits that he has spoken of things that he does not understand: 'Surely I spoke of things that I do not understand, things too wonderful for me to know ... My ears have heard of you but now my eyes *have seen you* therefore I despise myself and repent in dust and ashes' (Job 42: 3–6). He lived to be a 140 years old, his wealth was restored and he had 7 sons and 3 beautiful daughters. But, he had to suffer sickness first, then repent.

Instead of hearing about his god, he *saw* him. Here is the clue to the shift in understanding that occurs. This is the transcendence referred to in spirituality and the reason why some people see the purpose of suffering as a means of opening the heart to new meanings and direct experience. I am not recommending that we embrace suffering as a healing practice, it comes to us as an integral part of living anyway, only that the discernment of meaning in suffering is itself an achievement.

Miracles have been the exception. Their purpose is not simply evidential to convert others to the faith. When miracles are talked about in spiritual traditions, including the Christian Bible, those witnessing the miracle are asked to keep what they have seen to themselves. Miracles are instrumental for the person, like Job, being healed.

In the Christian tradition of healing we have accounts of an ancient practice of initiation by the spiritual teacher Jesus that are often taken literally at the expense of understanding their inner meaning. It is this lack of symbolic understanding that robs spiritual teachings of their potential for being understood, and thereby the achievement of transcendence for the perceiver.

Jesus and the blind man

We read earlier that Job had heard about his god. Then there was a change in understanding. He said that now he could see. This is a way of talking symbolically about a relationship with the divine that changes. A qualitatively different perception that can only be expressed metaphorically. If we take such stories literally we miss the point. The same applies in the story of the man blind from birth healed by Jesus (John 9).

As Jesus is going along with his disciples, he meets a man blind from birth. Like Job, he cannot see. He does not know his god in the same way that Job did not know. If we start from this premise, then the tale changes its meaning to one of spiritual instruction. The one who is *blind* sees the light of divine knowledge. The disciples ask Jesus if it is the man's fault that he is blind, or if it is the fault of his parents. The reply is that neither are at fault: the purpose is that 'the work of God might be displayed in his life' (John 9,v.3) and that it is his work to *enlighten* the man. The purpose of the teacher is to enlighten the man such that he sees.

Jesus then spits on the ground to make some mud and puts it on the man's eyes, telling him to go and wash in a pool. The man does this and can see. His neighbours are surprised at the change. He still appears the same outwardly, but is obviously inwardly different in demeanour. He no longer begs. They ask where Jesus is but he does not know.

This is a spiritual initiation. Through the mixture of 'earth', the ordinary stage of human knowledge, with spittle, the first part of the digestion process, an initiation is given by the teacher. Washing in 'water' is the stage of taking the man on to the path of spiritual knowledge leading to the divine by removing the mud of doubt through received knowledge, water. He now begins 'to see' having become enlightened by Jesus, who says earlier in the story that he is the light of the world. Shah (1990) explains this further as a series of stages in the process of initiation in Christian teaching where the first experience of baptism with water is followed with the Holy Spirit, air, and then with fire.

We have therefore a succession of stages in an ever-improving perception: from hearing to 'seeing', as in 'Do you see what I mean?'; not literally seeing as a sensory visual perception. This demonstrates the possibility of an inner knowledge within a religion, not simply the ritual aspects of the teaching. If Christian fundamentalists, of whatever persuasion, were really serious with externalist thinking then they would be going round spitting on the ground, smearing mud on the blind, sending patients to the nearest pond, wearing sandals and carrying satchels. Within religious texts there are codified hidden meanings by which they can be understood but to do so there has to be an interpreter who understands the code.

The story goes on. The man, newly enlightened, tells the local priests what has happened. They of course say that this is totally illegitimate because the person who has done this is not following their religious rules. When he says how it happened, they cannot believe it and ask him again. The healed man says that he told them once quite clearly; if they have not heard him the first time, then they are not likely to hear him the second. Of course, anyone challenging the knowledge of such hierarchies is thrown out straight away and accused of being a sinner, which is what happens in the story. It happened to the Klingbeils too; it happens in Churches and it happens in medicine.

But the tale is not yet at an end. When Jesus hears that the man has been thrown out by the priests, he asks him if he believes in 'The Son of Man' (John 9, v.35). The formerly blind man says he is willing to believe and is informed by Jesus with whom he is speaking. The man believes and worships him, whereupon Jesus tells him that the blind will see and those who see will become blind. Hearing this last statement, the priests ask if they too are blind. They are told that if they were blind then they are innocent, but claiming to know they are guilty.

This cannot then be a simple tale of healing the afflicted. It is an initiatory tale of bringing knowledge through contact. A story of enlightenment and the necessary change of perception that comes through spirituality.

If spiritual healing and prayer are about anything they are about this very change in a succession of changes. Focusing on the material is to miss the point. Furthermore, the tradition of miracles in varying faiths is that when a miracle is performed it is to remain hidden. The grounds being that miracles are of an extraordinary service and they are not done to make anyone happy or sad, nor to impress. Impressing people will only make them credulous and excited instead of learning something (Shah 1969).

Healing as a secondary ability

There is also a warning that accompanies the seekers of such healing powers, powers that are seen to be secondary to achieving spiritual knowledge. A spiritual seeker was talking to a teacher as she sat among her students. He said that through his studies and experiences he could walk on water. She told him, in return, that she could fly and that, if he so wished, they could have a private conversation in the air. He replied that sadly it would be impossible for him as he possessed no such powers of flight. She then told him that his power over water was something he shared with fish. The power over flying in the air can be done by any insect. Such abilities are no part of the real truth and may become the foundation of self-esteem and competitiveness, not spirituality (Shah 1971).

Many physicians testify that there are miraculous happenings in the field of health care, even if expressed as spontaneous remission. I am not simply talking about the miracle that nurses carry on their profession despite low status and poor pay. Such miracles of healing that we observe have different effects according to the stage of the observer. They challenge perceptions of the world and generate knowledge to those in need. Trying to explain them in terms of natural science and use them to justify prayer in healing is not going to help any of us. We need to discern the circumstances in which they occur and the purposes for those involved: thus the emphasis on healing narratives earlier, that cannot be contained in experimental studies, but can be included in qualitative research approaches (Aldridge 1998; Strauss and Corbin 1990).

Coda

The pursuit of evidence in support of prayer proves to be elusive. We continue to look in the wrong places, not recognizing its essentials, then declare that evidence does not exist. It offers another meaning to the concept of the 'double-blind' in clinical trials given the parable related above. If we are to submit prayer to a test, then we should at least be certain that the observations we will make incorporate the relevant criteria for assessing recovery.

What counts as a legitimate intervention and recognizable recovery using prayer in health-care delivery also has legal implications. I shall discuss this in the next chapter. We saw earlier that spirituality is the search for the divine and the achievement of unity. Prayer is the vehicle for this achievement. You can still pray with a broken leg. You cannot run with a broken leg. Knowing the difference between the two seems to be an elementary knowledge. The intention of prayer is to be with the divine, all other cares will fall away. For the sick, illness takes on a different meaning. It too may disappear. To look for a direct cause and effect with prayer is defying the spiritual teachings throughout the centuries as it fails to see the purposes of both sickness and prayer.

In terms of using medical practitioners, if you break a leg then an orthopaedic surgeon is the person to tell you exactly where the break is and to set the conditions appropriate for healing to take place. Once the optimal conditions are found, your body will heal itself, the original meaning of intentionality. What that exact process of healing entails is to be discovered. That the mind influences such healing is becoming apparent. This is an external knowledge of the world concerned with laws of cause and effect called science. There is also an internal knowledge that we have called spirituality. Both are important. Neither are to be neglected. Confusing prayer and its effects in the inappropriate world view helps no one. Learning its relationship to both heals. In both perspectives of knowledge, science and spirituality, attainment is achieved through teaching and guidance. If the world is given to us by the divine in all myriad of richness, then surely the blessings of medical knowledge and the dedication of its varying practitioners are provided by the same source.

7

Pluralism and treatment
Healing initiatives and authority

Once, when travelling on a ship, a young Italian came to me and said, 'I only believe in eternal matter.' I said, 'Your belief is not very different from my belief.' He was very surprised to hear a priest (he thought I was a priest) saying such a thing. He asked, 'What is your belief?' I said 'What you call eternal matter, I call eternal spirit. You call matter what I call spirit. What does it signify? It is only a difference in words. It is one Eternal.' (Inayat Khan 1974)

It would be wrong to permit medicine to use the authority it has gained from scientific and technical proficiency ... as a cloak to gain authority over questions that most in society consider moral and religious. (David Smolin 1995)

The true joy of every soul is in the realisation of the divine spirit; the absence of realisation keeps the soul in despair. (Inayat Khan 1979, p.105)

Healing today

During the twentieth century there were new calls for a healing revival from some church groups. This culminated within the last decade with a recognition of the Christian churches healing ministry (Courtenay 1991), albeit contentiously, and is often associated with a general interest in complementary medical initiatives calling for a consideration of the 'whole person'. There are also spiritual healing groups who have no church or religious affiliation and whose sole existence is the pursuit of spiritual healing.

Spiritual healing still exists throughout Western Europe (Sermeus 1987; Visser 1990) and occurs in two main forms. The first involves a hand contact, or near contact, between the healer and the patient. This is also seen in the church ritual of the laying on of hands. The second form is absent or distant healing where a healer or group of healers pray or meditate for the patient who is absent from their presence. Patients can be far removed from the healing group. Healers emphasize that a special state of mind is required for this influence to occur.

Older 'shamanistic techniques' of healing have mainly died out in Europe except for remote rural areas in the north (Vaskilampi 1990). Shamans, present in most tribal cultures throughout the world, are an elite who use techniques of ecstasy (dream and trance) to cure people, guard the soul of the community and direct its religious life (Eliade 1989). While trances are used to cure, they are also a means of transporting souls to other worlds and mediating between humans and gods. The recruitment of such healers is by inheritance or spiritual vocation, entails an arduous apprenticeship and an initiatory crisis that involves the novice shaman being cured of a sickness. Any such notions of modern-day healers as shamans is a rather misguided romantic fantasy revealing more about the healers' need for power and reward than the role of healer in present day culture (see Table 7.1).

The personal quest emphasized by the modern-day spiritual healer is incompatible with the service to the community which the shaman provides; nor is there the validity offered by the community for such practice. There is a long apprenticeship and the initiatory crisis is indeed hard. Perhaps junior medical practitioners with their extended apprenticeship after the initiatory crisis of getting a place at medical school, the extended hours of overtime in early practice and their kinship ties, coming from medical families, meet the criteria best. That they go on to take the medicines, in terms of drug abuse, as Sonneck and Wagner (1996) suggest is yet another supporting argument for medical practitioner as modern-day shaman. However, probably the originators of Alcoholics Anonymous, with their emphasis on the dry alcoholic in his telling in a communal gathering, come closer to the spirit of the shamanistic ideal.

The idea of a crisis alone as initiatory must be taken with care, as emotional breakdown and subsequent indoctrination are the basis of conditioning techniques. In conjunction with conformist behaviour we have the basis for bigotry. Some groups claim to be spiritual healers, but in reality are exercising their need for emotional satisfaction, excitement and control and neglect the needs of patients. The code of conduct offered by the National Federation of Spiritual Healers (NFSH 1999) is a useful guide for ascertaining the validity of such healing approaches.

Table 7.1 Differences between health practitioners, modern spiritual healers and traditional shamans

Health practitioner	Modern spiritual healer	Traditional shaman
Self-selection to a professional group, although medicine runs in families.	Self-selection often to a group, or by nomination within a hierarchy.	Selection by crisis or inheritance.
No initiatory crisis, pathological crisis a hindrance to vocational training.	No initiatory crisis necessary, but concept of 'wounded healer' plays an important role.	Initiatory crisis sign of vocation, pathological crisis necessary for vocation.
Personal quest acceptable.	Personal quest valued.	Personal quest devalued or irrelevant.
Institutional training.	No institutional training necessary.	No institutional training.
No arduous mental and physical ordeal.	No arduous mental and physical ordeal.	Arduous mental and physical ordeal.
Limited apprenticeship.	Brief apprenticeship.	Long apprenticeship.
Legitimacy bestowed by institution on behalf of the community (licensing).	Legitimacy bestowed by community.	Legitimacy bestowed by community.
No kinship ties.	No kinship ties.	Kinship ties.
Variable status.	Low status.	High status.
Patient removed from environment, often treated behind closed doors, with the focus on individuals or dyads (rarely as family or social groups).	Patient removed from environment, often treated behind closed doors, with the focus on individuals or dyads (rarely as family or social groups).	Patient treated within the community as public phenomenon.
Patient is the agent of their own healing and responsible.	Spiritual forces or energy channelled by the healer is the agency of healing, patient responsible.	The shaman is the agent of cure and responsible for the results.
The patient takes the drugs.	The patient receives the healing.	The shaman takes the drugs.
There are time restraints to consultation.	There are flexible time restraints to consultation.	No time restraints to consultation.
For the individual good of the patient.	For the individual good of the patient.	For the social good of the community.
For the material or personal gain of the therapist.	For the material, personal or spiritual benefit of the therapist.	A sacred event for the community with no personal benefit.

How spiritual healing is explained, its influence demonstrated and evidence presented raises a number of problems. First, that which is of the 'spirit', non-material, is not readily accessible to demonstration and explanation within the parameters of a physicalist science, although matter is influenced. Second, the words used for describing differing forms of healing are based on varying traditions and have differing meanings, although for some spiritual teachers the difference in a belief in eternal matter and a belief in eternal spirit is one of a difference in words alone. Third, the very search for definition is antithetical to the spiritual endeavour. As scientists we want precision and to know exactly. In the search for spiritual understanding, it is the openness of the question, a question that asserts itself over and over again, that is important. The vocation to seek the divine has no formula by which it can be achieved.

We surely find the same problem with health in terms of becoming whole. A single definition eludes us. With each altered definition there are different ramifications for different stages in our lives as we saw in Chapter 4. Each definition will be personal. The search for meaning is a personal quest revealing a subjective knowledge predicated upon an individual development in consciousness. That definition has a certain validity when it is achieved as a life lived to the full. Life is dynamic, there is a necessary performance that is convincing. It is rarely what we say we are that convinces others, it is how we treat them and what we do that gains validity. The valid and the vital are intertwined.

Who is to know what is true?

Away from the privacy of the individual search, we live together with others and share a common language that enables us to convey our understandings to each other and from one generation to the next. This is the work of culture. The social is important. In relationships we learn about ourselves. We all need a friend.

We also have obligations to others. The social is what is common to all religions offering forms for experiencing nature and the divine. Achieving truth is a social activity dependent upon its embodiment in individuals. Culture offers religious forms in symbols, language and ritual localized for temporal and geographical contexts whereby that truth can be expressed, individuals protected and behaviour regulated. The same goes for science and secular knowledge where we have various forms and means of ascertaining the truth and realizing the presence of a greater unity. This realization also protects communities and regulates behaviour. Only when we lose the concept of unity, or fail to achieve it, is the ecology broken.

Such a relative and liberal perspective, however, soon brings charges of heresy from the conservativisms of both religious traditions and scientific medicine where there are fixed hierarchies, (each tradition has its priesthood), for determining what is believable and how evidence is to be sought for those beliefs.

Indeed, the Gnostic tradition of a personal knowledge of god has challenged the authority of the priesthood as mediators of spiritual knowledge. So too today, we have a similar situation where knowledge of healing by consumers challenges the authority of those charged with health-care delivery. Alternative practitioners and laity are making challenges to be licensed to heal (Aldridge 1986). In addition, medical authority is also being challenged in terms of responsibility in health care (May 1995) and to what extent religion has a part to play in debates surrounding medial ethics (Orr and Genesen 1998; Savulescu 1998).

Yet built into modern medicine is a religious foundation of thinking. We saw in Chapter 3 how Asklepios, son of Apollo, symbolizes a unity of medicine and religion and some of his children represent personifications of the healing powers. The Hippocratic Corpus that represents the body of work underpinning the development of medical ethics also reflects a religious background to medicine. The Hippocratic oath is a document swearing allegiance to 'Apollo Physician and Asceplias and Hygieia and Panakeia and all the gods and goddesses, making them my witness' (Smolin 1995).

While there may be moves towards a secular scientific ethic in medicine, it is hardly likely that such a secular ethic yet exists. Medical ethics are clearly based on religious grounds. Nor is it likely to change given that the application of medical ethics implicates issues about the alleviation of suffering, the preservation of life and the withdrawal of treatment.

We are currently faced with the ability to change the genetic structure of living beings whereupon we have obtained the keys to creation. If these decisions become solely secular, based on the priorities of technological innovation and commercial exploitation, then we will have abandoned ourselves to the lowest of human forces. This is not an anti-technology argument, nor is it against the understanding of the possibilities for gene manipulation in medicine, rather that those understandings are made within a broader context of human ethics.

Religious perspectives are important. The essence of the religious is an understanding of what it is to be human within the ecology of nature in relationship to the divine. While we must utilize the understandings that we glean from medical science, those understandings need to be allied to a broader perspective concerned with the meaning of life and death. Such understandings, as we saw in Chapters 2 and 3, are predicated on the religious and discerned through the spiritual. The medical can be informed by the religious, both are united by a spiritual search for meaning.

Healing practice and ethics of treatment

With practitioners and patients interested in prayer, there is a concern about how such a therapeutic approach can be incorporated into clinical practice. Such concerns are about the licensing of practitioners, the quality of qualifications, the protection of patients and providing evidence for treatment. These arguments are also about protecting professional practice from 'ousiders' and restricting access to health-care funding. There is a territory of practice to be defended and a living to be made out of healing and many arguments are about access, or its restriction, to this professional territory.

Magaletta and Brawer (1996) remind us that therapists are ethically bound to practise and provide only those services for which they are qualified by education, training and experience. If this is so, they ask whether or not therapists are taught how to pray and what texts would be used. Traditional teachings, authorized ritualized practices and hierarchies of practitioners would be rejected by many New Age groups as authoritarian and, as we saw in Chapter 5, would be definitely regarded as 'churchy'. Similarly, if in traditional systems what comes from the spirit is given freely, as grace, then it is for no one to charge for such services. Indeed, if patients recover through prayer to demonstrate healing abilities, then surely the intercessors should be paying the patients for validating their work.

Guidelines for practice in England

In England various spiritual healing organizations and some religious groups have formed themselves into a confederation of healing organizations so that they can practise in hospitals and take referrals from physicians. This confederation issues strict guidelines for practice and conduct (NFSH 1999) which have been worked out with the help of the British Medical Association and the varying Royal Colleges. The code of conduct covers legal obligations, how to handle the relationship with the patient regarding medical treatment and emphasizes full co-operation with medical authorities. There are clear guidelines for healers visiting hospitals which include instructions about not wearing white coats, how to behave on the ward and how to obtain permission from the nursing officer. Unlike doctors, healers must disclaim an ability to cure but offer to attempt to heal in some measure, without any promise of recovery, and behave with courtesy, discretion and tact. If healing should take place in such stringent conditions of psychological pessimism regarding cure, then criticisms that these methods rely on 'patient suggestibility' must surely be found wanting. Similarly, we might ask ourselves, how doctors would compare given the same restrictions and comparable injunctions to behave with tact and courtesy.

Patients are advised to see a doctor concerning their condition. If a doctor refers a patient, then the doctor remains clinically responsible. The healer must not countermand instructions or any treatments prescribed by a doctor and diagnosis remains the responsibility of the doctor. Under no circumstances must the healer give a diagnosis to the patient. As we saw in the studies by Brown (1995), Brown and Sheldon (1989) and Dixon (1998), some general practitioners have responded favourably to such guidelines and make regular referrals to spiritual healers.

There are also legal considerations to be made regarding confidentiality, consent for treatment, the treatment of children under the age of eighteen and the dispensing of herbal remedies. There are special regulations concerning the notification of sexually transmitted disease. It is illegal to practise dentistry without qualification and an offence to attend a woman in childbirth other than in an emergency.

These guidelines exemplify a tolerant politic of health-care practice. Medical practitioners utilize the science base of their health-care training and understanding, but also have resort to a broader perspective of knowledge. Furthermore, this knowledge base is not simply that of the doctor, it is becoming a knowledge base that both share. However, we see in the ways that these rules are formulated that no matter how much practitioners emphasize the scientific and the secular, the symbolic comes to the fore in proscriptions regarding clothing, speech and behaviour.

Medical alternatives and the law

Frohock (1993) alerts us to the problems surrounding health-care delivery, the regulation of medical practices and political power in a liberal society like the USA when there are competing beliefs about the nature of reality; that is, who decides what medical treatments, conventional or complementary, are valid. His argument centres around cases that highlight the freedom of choice issues surrounding specific therapies where a life is at stake and the competence of the individual to select a particular, perhaps unconventional, therapy that is questioned by the state. For example, who is to decide the appropriate therapy for a child whose life is threatened by an illness that demands urgent treatment? The state or the parent? Essentially the individual freedom of the parent can be challenged, in the case of minors, by the state if a treatment is chosen that is not authorized and supervised by one of its own licensed practitioners. This liberal dilemma brings to our attention a matter that demands urgent debate in a modern world where the established orthodoxies of medicine and religion are being questioned (Bullis 1991; Merrick 1994; Smolin 1995; Tavolaro 1991).

Legal examples surrounding treatment controversies relating to competence are of profound importance. These cases raise not only important issues of state involvement and individual freedom, but also what medical initiatives are acceptable and what evidence is valid for treatment prognosis when priorities must be established among competing healing claims. A 12-year-old Tennessee girl suffering from cancer has to be treated medically, even though her father opposes treatment on religious grounds. A child is withdrawn prematurely by his parents from a chemotherapy programme against the wishes of the attending physician to begin a nutritional treatment regime and a New York court mandates the child's return to conventional therapy. Reading the varying perspectives from the participants of such dramas, we see that the acceptance of what counts as evidence about which treatment decisions can be made in the field of healing, both conventional and alternative, is a matter of political negotiation. To decide in such cases of conflict between parents and practitioner demands a special moral skill on behalf of the arbitrators as both sets of beliefs have equal power.

The case of baby Rena (Smolin 1995) exemplifies the issues at stake when the belief systems collide. Here the medical ethics of the physician to provide relief for the distress of his patient and attempt no cure when disease has mastery, knowing that everything is not possible in medicine, collide with the fundamentalist beliefs of a couple who demand aggressive treatment in the conviction that a miracle will occur to justify their faith.

Baby Rena was born infected with AIDS and her mother gave her over to state care. She was adopted when four months old by an evangelical Christian couple who believed that, after prayer, through nurturing her they would be a testimony to the body of Christ. This was not simply providing love to a dying child but spiritual warfare against the AIDS disease and would use the principles of the Bible, prayer and faith to provide a miraculous healing.

Within two weeks she was placed on a respirator suffering with pneumonia and the physicians thought she would die. The couple prayed. Rena recovered. The parents claimed a miracle and the physicians a medical success. Neither appeared to consider that it was a combination of the two that called for and sent the boat of recovery.

At nine months Rena was healthy enough to go home to her foster parents where she lived until she was fifteen months old. Again she was hospitalized and placed on a respirator. Rena required increasing doses of medication to keep her from becoming agitated and thrashing about in pain. The physician, who had taken over responsibility for the treatment, believed that the respirator should be removed, that the child was suffering, in pain, and there was no hope. However, Rena's parents wanted aggressive medical treatment. Her physician was concerned that although Rena might live for months on a respirator, the only way to relieve her pain was to sedate her so much that there was no purpose in living. She was sure to die.

Rena's foster father objected that this was a decision which only God could take and she should remain on the respirator. An ethical committee was convened to discuss the case with the parents. When a decision to take unilateral action was dismissed by the hospital attorney, the foster father took this as 'an act of God' (Smolin 1995, p.965).

After two weeks on the respirator, Rena breathed on her own. The parents proclaimed a miracle. When Rena's condition soon deteriorated again, her physician wanted her to die in her parents' arms with decency and comfort, not with infusions and breath being pumped mechanically in and out of her. Her parents refused. They wanted faith to be illustrated in action, as if taking a child in one's arms and allowing her to die in peace is not action enough. Rena died that afternoon, despite the respirator and the treatment. Her foster mother was informed by telephone.

The parents belonged to a church which embraces the view that God intends all believers to be healthy, if they will only 'claim' such health. When taken literally this is a religious view, it is possibly a magical view and is not a spiritual view. However, in a truly postmodern sense, Rena's parents converted the injunction of their church's ideology, that usually deprecates medical care as a lack of faith, and sought maximum medical care, in the context of which a miracle would occur. Yet in seeking this care, they rejected its very essence in the advice of its practitioners. Divorced from a faith, where Rena would have died lovingly but quickly, and a scientific epistemology, where Rena would have died lovingly and comfortably, they pursued a headlong course of faithfully committed superstition where Rena died anyway, intubated and separate from her foster parents.

The tragedy is that the physicians, the hospital chaplain and the parents could not find a way to enter into dialogue, other than conflict. We have to ask ourselves how much others must suffer to maintain our own belief systems intact through dogma. As Smolin remarks, 'Religious freedom does not require that religion be above questioning or dialogue' (p.995). The challenge for us all is how to promote a dialogue when world views collide – for surely here is the root of healing.

While the arena of this discussion has so far been mainly confined to the tragic cases of children, the debate will be further widened when claims to validity are made for alternative medicines if its practitioners are licensed by the state to practise.

A major conflict arises when two seemingly opposing realities meet. Religious groups of varying denominations emphasize that healing, often through the agency of prayer, can occur by faith, supernatural agency or living in the correct manner. One particular group, that of Christian Science, emphasizes that illness is the product of an incorrect state of mind, that God created everything perfect and anything less than that is a lie about creation. Correction of this flawed state, bringing thought into accord with reality, leads to a return to health. The reality in this instance is being in accord with God and may stand in conflict with a mortal material reality. As modern medicine has its practitioners, then so too does Christian Science, although such practitioners are not licensed either by the state or by the Church of Christ Scientist itself. When a child is ill then Christian Scientists can call upon such a practitioner to minister to them through counselling and prayer. This decision does not necessarily preclude modern conventional medicine. A doctor may be consulted to establish the exact material conditions for which the spiritual ministration must be found and to hedge against charges of negligence in the case of children (May 1995). However, the expectancy of the Church is that parents who take such a path will eventually see the error of their ways and return to the fold. It is the consequence of consultation with a medical practitioner that is the source of potential conflict when the physician recognizes an illness that demands urgent medical treatment. A child may be 'dangerously ill' and the parents reluctant to accede to a conventional medical treatment recommendation. Indeed, recommendation in such cases of urgency becomes a demand. In such a situation, the fundamental right of parents to rear their children free of government intervention is not absolute.

The fact that there are varying schools of medical practice and beliefs other than the orthodox is accepted in American law. John Baumgartner was treated at his own request for acute prostatitis by a Christian Science practitioner and a Christian Science nurse. Ten days elapsed before he died. No medical doctor was called in. He was a wealthy industrialist and bequeathed one-half of his estate to the Christian Science church. His family objected and brought a wrongful death action against the church, the practitioner and the nurse. However, the court dismissed the case for medical malpractice on the ground that one form of medical practice cannot be judged by the criteria of another form of medical practice. In this case Christian Science practitioners were using spiritual means, not medical aid. The patient had specifically requested Christian Science treatment when he became ill, despite advice during his illness to seek medical aid, and could not have reasonably have expected anything other than spiritual healing (Tammelleo 1986).

In Chapter 1, I argue for a pluralistic society where there are alternate explanations of reality. By making judgements about what is legitimate health care we enter into the complex world of decision making and responsibility. Lives may be at stake. Individual freedom has limitations in civil society. Deciding on what those limitations are is a matter of continuing debate and compromise and centres around the notion of authority.

Authority

As we have seen in Chapters 3 and 4, the role of religious and medical authority is increasingly being questioned by consumers and users. Where authority is understood as an expert role of guidance, then there is tolerance. Where that role extends into restricting what another person can do, then we see continuing rejection. People are no longer willing to accept traditional authority structures or the knowledge contained within them. In religion, 'God said' is rejected; so too with the all-encompassing statements of medical science. Ethnic, religious, minority, linguistic groups are all demanding that their perspectives and interpretations of the truth are heard. This is the nature of pluralism and the postmodern plethora of voices. It encourages a variety of forms of expression but can militate against coherence. New authorities regarding health understandings and belief systems appear. The user is faced with a bewildering choice. If we look at the advice regarding healthy eating and nutrition then we could starve waiting for sensible coherent advice. We have to learn to choose and those choices need to be informed. This demands discriminatory knowledge; not simply a plethora of information but a means of discerning what is necessary for practice and therefore a responsible education.

The foundation of the New Age myth (Hanegraaff 1999) is that of an un-limited spiritual evolution in which the self learns from its experiences, experiences themselves that are self-constructed. As we saw in Chapter 4, individuals construct their own identities and one of the elements by which an identity is constructed is 'spiritual'. Individual treatment regimes, 'growth' practices and techniques of self-realization are related to fitness and health and described as lifestyles. From such perspectives, healing is concerned not with restricting us to a one-dimensional sense of being according to an accepted orthodox world view, but the possibility for the interpretation of the self as new. This possibility of a new interpretation is the foundation on which the recovering alcoholic builds his life.

Some like-minded individuals form groups for mutual support. These groups reject authoritarian religious approaches and emphasize a radical symbolic perspective that embeds itself in a secular culture. The same process can be observed in attitudes towards health care and towards science and technology. Hanegraaff (1999, p.149) argues that this secular pluralist approach in contem-porary society is not based upon science but popular mythologies of science. If this is so, then we need a system of education that emphasizes discernment in scientific thinking such that individuals have the resources to inform themselves. The same can be said regarding spirituality. This topos is a search for knowledge.

The negative side of a self-informed, constructivist approach is a rampant narcissism and a question is raised about finding a place for common moral values when the individual is always placed to the fore.

Research in healing

Medical professionals are becoming aware that there are aspects of health which do not fall within their range of knowledge. For those elements to be incorp-orated into practice, a realm of clinical evidence is being demanded that is quite inappropriate. I am not saying that spirituality and its influence on health-care practices should be accepted simply because it is a good idea, rather that the means of gathering and displaying evidence is discussed.

Critics have found the strict methodology of natural science is often wanting when applied to the study of human health-care behaviour (Aldridge and Pietroni

1987; Burkhardt and Kienle 1980, 1983). This critique has stimulated calls for innovation in clinical medical research and therapy (Aldridge 1992, 1996; Reason and Rowan 1981). A significant factor in the desire for innovation is a growing awareness by doctors of the importance of a patient's social and cultural milieu and a recognition that the health beliefs of a patient and understandings of personal meanings should be incorporated in treatment. What we need in clinical research is a discipline that seeks to discover methods which express clinical changes as they occur in the individual, rather than methods which reflect a group average. How clinical change occurs and is recognized will depend upon not only the view of the researcher and clinician, but also upon the beliefs and understandings of the patients and their families (Aldridge 1998).

There is often a split in medical science between researchers and clinicians. Researchers see themselves as rational and rigorous in their thinking and tend to regard clinicians as sentimental and biased, which in turn elicits comments from clinicians about inhuman treatment and reductionist thinking. We are faced with the problem of how to promote in clinical practice research that has scientific validity in terms of rigour and, at the same time, a clinical validity for the patient and clinician.

The randomized trial appears to be theoretically relevant for the clinical researcher, but has all too often randomized away what should be specifically relevant for the clinician and patient. A comparative trial of two chemotherapy regimes assumes that the treatment or control groups to which patients are randomly assigned contain evenly balanced populations. What is sought from such a trial is that one method works significantly better than another comparing group averages. Yet as clinicians we want to know what method works best for the individual patient. Our interest lies not in the group average, but with those patients who do well with such treatment and those who do not respond so well. Furthermore, the randomizing of patients with specific prognostic factors obscures therapeutic effect. Rather than searching for a non-specific chemo-therapy treatment of a particular cancer, we may be better advised to seek out those factors which allow us to deliver a specific treatment for recognized individuals with a particular cancer. This is not to argue against randomization exclusively, rather that we have randomized the patient rather than the treatment. As Weinstein says:

> Randomisation tends to obscure rather than illuminate, interactive effects between treatments and personal characteristics. Thus if Treatment A is best for one type of patient and Treatment B is best for another type, a randomised study would only be able to indicate which treatment performs best overall. If we wanted to discover the effect on subgroups, one would have to separate out the variable anyway. (Weinstein 1974, p.1281)

We may well say the same of the non-specific use of prayer, we do not know the use of prayer already by the patient in a group, nor those praying for her. Nor do we know at what stage that person is in terms of suffering such that prayer will bring not only relief but an new understanding. Prayer is not like a medication, as yet no dose response formula has been discovered.

Science and medicine: What science does not know

Modern science implies that there is a common map of the territory of healing, with particular co-ordinates and given symbols for finding our way around, which is the map of scientific medicine. We need to recognize that scientific medicine emphasizes one particular way of knowing among others. Scientific thinking maintains the myth that to know anything we must be scientists. However, people who live in vast desert areas find their way across those trackless terrains without any understandings of scientific geography. They also know the pattern of the weather without recourse to what we know as the science of meteorology.

In a similar way, people know about their own bodies and have understandings about their own lives without the benefit of anatomy or psychology. Furthermore, people know of their own god or connection to a higher power without the benefits of an elaborated theology as we saw in Chapter 5. They may not confer the same meanings on their experiences of health and illness as we researchers do, yet it is towards an understanding of personal and idiosyncratic beliefs that we might most wisely be guiding our research endeavours. By understanding the stories people tell us of their healing and the insights this brings, we may begin truly to understand the efficacy of prayer. That health and the divine are brought together in such spiritualities is a challenge for renewal of our understanding in health care, not a ground for dismissal as invalid.

When we speak of scientific or experimental validity, we speak of a validity that has to be conferred by a person or group of persons on the work or actions of another group. This is a 'political' process. With the obsession for 'objective truths' in the scientific community other 'truths' are ignored. As clinicians we have many ways of knowing: by intuition, through experience and by observation. If we disregard these 'knowings' then we promote the idea that there is an objective definitive external truth which exists as 'tablets of stone' and that only we, the initiated, have access to it. This criticism applies also to the dogma of religion that refuses to consider what other evidence the world provides. Simply saying that the world is evil will not resolve the need of the necessary dialogue for transcending seemingly opposing views.

The people with whom clinicians work in the therapist–patient relationship are not experimental units. Nor are the measurements made on these people separate and independent sets of data. While at times it may be necessary to treat the data as independent of the person, we must be aware that we are doing this. Otherwise when we come to measure particular personal variables we face many complications. Consider a person like George in Chapter 1 who has been treated unsuccessfully for chronic leukaemia with a bone marrow transplant. The clinical measurements of blood status, weight and temperature are important. However, they belong to a different realm of understanding from issues of anxiety about the future, the experience of pain, the anticipation of personal and social losses and the existential feeling of abandonment. These defy comparative measurement. Yet if we are to investigate therapeutic approaches to chronic disease, we need to investigate these subjective and qualitative realms. While we may be able to make little change in blood status, we can take heed of emotional status and propose initiatives for treatment. The goal of therapy is not always to cure, it can also be to comfort and relieve. The involvement of the physician with the biologic dimension of disease has resulted in an amnesia for the necessary understanding of suffering in the patient (Cassell 1991).

In the same way, we can achieve changes in existential states through prayer and meditation, the evidence for which can only be metaphorically expressed and humanly witnessed. Are we to impoverish our culture by denying that this happens and discounting what people tell us? What then are we to trust in our lives, the dialogue with our friends or the displays of our machines? This is not an argument against technology. It is an argument for narrative and relationship in understanding what it is to be human.

In terms of outcomes measurement, we face further difficulties. The people we see in our clinics do not live in isolation. Life is rather a messy laboratory and continually influences the subjects of our therapeutic and research endeavours. The way people respond in situations is sometimes determined by the way in which they have understood the meaning of that situation. The meaning of hair loss, weight loss, loss of potency, loss of libido, impending death and the nature of suffering will be differently perceived in varying cultures. To this balding, aging researcher, hair loss is a fact of life. My Greek neighbour says that if it happens to him it will be a disaster. When we deliver a powerful therapeutic agent we are not treating an isolated example of a clinical entity, but intervening in an ecology of responses and beliefs which are somatic, psychological, social and spiritual. Indeed the whole notion of 'placebo' is based upon the ability of belief to exert an influence.

In a similar way, what Western medicine understands as surgery, intubation and medication, others may perceive as mutilation, invasion and poisoning. Cultural differences regarding the integrity of the body will influence ethical issues such as abortion and body transplants. Treatment initiatives may be standardized in terms of the culture of the administering researchers, but the perceptions of the subjects of the research and their families may be incongruous and various. Actually, we know from studies of treatment options in breast cancer that physicians' beliefs also vary, and these beliefs influence the information which they give to their patients (Ganz 1992).

When we have to take decisions regarding the prolongation of life we are not solely engaged in secular matters. As we saw earlier, the physician treating baby Rena knew what the technological limitations were of the scientific medicine that he practised and what was necessary for him as a compassionate physician to encourage for the patient in his care to fulfil his Hippocratic oath.

Difficulties in researching prayer and spiritual healing

From what we have read so far there are major difficulties with healing research:

1. Achieving transcendence, an understanding of purpose and meaning as a performed identity, is an activity. It occurs in a relationship which is informed by culture. Research initiatives that concentrate on the healer fail to understand the activity of the patient, lose sight of the relationship and ignore the cultural factors involved. I am using culture here to refer to the system of symbolic meanings that is available, not demographic data. Losing this nesting of contexts fragments the healing endeavour, emphasizing a passive patient that receives healing rather than an active patient participating in a common enterprise.

2. Much research is carried out using a traditional medical science paradigm but the intention of that research is not made clear. If the intention is to demonstrate the efficacy of spiritual healing approaches and prayer, then the methodology is clearly misguided. I suspect that much of this research is not being carried out for patients but as a strategy in the politics of establishing alternative healing initiatives within conventional medical approaches. Therefore we have healing groups promoting their own interest and adopting the methodological approach of randomized clinical trials considered to be suitable for acceptance, rather than looking at what is necessary for discovering what is happening. This is not to say that the results of clinical randomized trials are not influential, rather that they are limited in their applicability as far as prayer and healing are to be understood if (a) the patient is expected to be active; (b) there has to be a relationship with the healer; (c) there are no definite end-points in time; (d) healing can

appear as differing phenomena; (e) the prayer has to be no-specific and non-directional.[1]

3. Healing, like prayer, is not an homogeneous practice and is not susceptible to standardization. Attempts at standardization would no longer make it prayer but superstitious incantation or magical hand passes.

4. The ability to heal is seen in some traditions as a divine gift. It may not be available to everyone and even those who have the gift find it is not available all the time. Ascertaining who has the ability and when is not easy. Healing is also considered, in some traditions, to be a secondary ability of spiritual development that can be systematically applied, but it is an advanced ability. This again proves to be a difficulty, as presumably there are more practitioners with lower abilities than advanced practitioners who are more reliable in their efficacy. Who in the world of healing practitioners is going to say that they are less advanced? Those who are advanced in such understandings will probably see no need to subject such knowledge to material worldly proof.

Indeed, we must return to the purpose of proof. We see already that spiritual healing is practised and that medical practitioners refer to such healers. If the grounds of research are for payment or to institute professional practice, then maybe the results will be elusive than when the purpose is for the pursuit and improvement of human knowledge. One system of knowledge cannot be predicated on proofs from another system of knowledge.

Spirituality, as we saw in Chapter 1, is one way of achieving truth. It stands alongside science. We do not have to be desperate in trying to fit both into the same mould. The challenge is to reconcile both in a greater understanding of the truth. That is transcendence.

Narrative and the possibility of change

Gergen states that: 'The point of these therapies is not so much to cure the individual as to develop forms of viable meaning' (1997, p.27). When people come to their practitioners they are asking about what will become of them. What will their future be like? Will there be a change? Some practitioners make a prognosis based on the interview that they have had with the patient. Sometimes this will be the dreaded answer to the question, 'How long do I have to live?' But with each interview there is the question of when healing will take place. What

---

[1] The concept of 'Thy will be done' as an effective form of prayer, following Dossey (1993), ruins a one-tailed statistical test.

can be expected in the near future and is there any hope of a cure. The story of what happens is, in part, a clinical history. It is also no less than the narration of destiny, the unfolding of a person's life purpose (Larner 1998). When we talk with the dying, this sense of purpose, 'Was it all worthwhile?', is a critical moment in coping with the situation.

Narratives are the recounting of what happens in time. They are not simply located in the past, but are also about real events that happen now and what expectations there are for the future. The teller of the narrative is an active agent. She is not passively experiencing her past but performing an identity with another person. That other person, as doctor, priest or healer, has the moral obligation through the therapeutic contract to listen and engage in the healing relationship. Narratives are told. This performance aspect is what gives a narrative vitality and instructs us, as listeners, to what we must attend (Aldridge 1996). Narratives are not simply private accounts that we relate to ourselves. They have a public function and will vary according to whom is listening and the way in which the listeners are reacting. Qualitative research has incorporated such narratives into its approach to understanding health care (Aldridge 1998; Hall 1998; Strauss and Corbin 1990; van Manen 1998).

Change is concerned with how the future meets the past and how we make sense of such a transition. In narratives there is the possibility to open up to something new. This is where the potential for healing takes place and where we can introduce hope, the moment that transcends what has gone before. Scientific probability assumes that the future is predicated on the past; it is the fatal as opposed to the transcendental. Fate is the necessity that follows the past. It is the basis of scientific reasoning that informs prospective clinical studies and is as much a belief as the hope for a different future. Destiny, however, assumes some purpose other than the statistics of probability. Narratives bring a coherence and order to life stories. Stories make sense. Yet the scientific null hypothesis assumes, at the very core of its reasoning, that there is no such coherence (Larner 1998). Technology strives to domesticate time as *chronos*, to make time even and predictable. In an earlier book (Aldridge 1996), I wrote of time as *kairos*, uneven, biological and decisive, in that the moment must be seized. This makes a mockery of fixed outcomes in that the time and logic of healing may have modes elusive to commercialized requirements of health-care delivery. Peace of mind may occur but no cure. Forgiveness may take place but no change in survival time. Are we really to throw away such outcomes of peace of mind and forgiveness because they find no immediate material expression? Perhaps it is the very denial of those qualities that provokes the restlessness of people today as they seek an elusive state of health despite the material riches of Western cultures.

When we consider narratives about the future we construct possible life courses based upon our own agency. Of course there is a link to the past, but we have the possibility for transcending the past. Hope is what lifts us out of that moment to new possibilities. We choose the people with whom that narrative will be told in the future. We choose the people who will influence that narrative. Agency in this sense is the ability to shift between the principles under which life is lived and the potential discourses that will be used to describe such a life. This does not mean that the dying will escape death. But the narrative of dying that we make, how dying is performed, with whom we die and how that dying is remembered are important. Hope lies in the ability to perform such a narrative.

If we consider the processes of palliative care, then we see that patients actively choose the medical initiatives they want during that process, and often in collaboration with their loved ones. The dignity of dying is a narrative for the patient and one that will be recounted by the survivors. This is exactly what disturbs the lives of the survivors remaining after suicide. There is no healing narrative in which the survivor can take part. It is difficult to transcend the past narrative because an important person is lacking.

Accepting death

Dying is a process that occurs in time and within a social context of significant others. Within this time trajectory our identity is threatened, as are those with whom we live and are loved. The move from wife to widow, from healthy hopeful to sick and dying patient is a challenge, so too for the professional carers. Their identities are challenged by the nature of their healing endeavours as successful or failing.

My brother-in-law died recently. He had Hodgkin's disease and was treated with radiotherapy and several courses of chemotherapy. In the end he died as a result of the treatment. His digestive system was debilitated through the radiotherapy, a known side effect. In the last days he was taken into hospital as he became progressively weaker, and eventually into intensive care. Despite the clear evidence of his impending and imminent death, he was aggressively intubated to drain his abdomen. After his death, the intubations were explained as necessary to show that all possible had been done. But to what end? Surely not for the patient but for the practitioners to maintain faith in a technological medicine that by then had failed and to maintain their identities as successful healers and the success rate of the hospital ward. For his siblings and his partner it was an unnecessary intervention that prevented him dying in peace, ignoring his literal last requests.

When death is not accepted then we see the worst excesses of technological intervention where the patient and practitioners lose all dignity. We have to work to meet the challenge of maintaining identities in changing situations both by the patients, their families and those implementing treatment. Within the trajectory of dying there are 'points of option' where decisions have to be made (Baszanger

1998). This work is action and through this action in a social context we have the chance for new meanings to be gleaned.

When we consider chronic degenerative disease, while there may be little hope in the diagnosis, there may be hope in the ensuing narrative for the sufferer and her family if we allow for meanings that transcend current understandings. I am not talking here about cure but about healing. By increasing the variety of points of option in a narrative we have more opportunities for transcendence to take place. The narratives that we have are our biographies and these biographies take place within a body. In chronic disease this biography is interrupted in a way which we had not planned. The body will then play an important part in any narrative constructions of identity. Bodies have their narratives and they perform their corporeality in the cultural contexts of healing encounters.

Some spiritual healers encourage the negligence of the body as it is only a vehicle for the spirit and its impulses must be denied. This is an incredibly limited view of spirituality. Furthermore, as we saw in Chapter 4, spirituality as it is performed by the body is a vital aspect of health identities. While mind–body medicine has emphasized the incorporation of mind into the argument, there is no reason to leave out the body and generate a mind–mind medicine. The body may have its reasons that reason does not know. Knowing what is mind, what is body, and the wisdom to know the difference between the two is perhaps an important step in our coming health-care understandings. That spirit unites them is another.

Relationship as central

Healing encounters are part of the social world and are with other embodied individuals. 'Being for the other' is an essentially creative activity involving the sensual body against the rational impulses of totalitarianism (Shilling and Mellor 1998). Shilling and Mellor see modern society as dehumanizing because it fails to grasp the emotional responses necessary for 'being for the other'. Modernity is based upon control, with a distance placed between the observer and events. In a socially responsible healing culture, this distance must be replaced. We are literally being asked to 'be there' by the other, and to be there in a sensual relationship that will entail a lived body. While it may be necessary for those working in intensive care who treated my brother-in-law to protect themselves from contact with the other as a means of survival, then we must consider what the ramifications are for patient care. If the emotional responses necessary for understanding the process of treatment in the context of dying are lacking, then we must question the quality of that care for patients and practitioners. Given the high rates of stress within the healing profession, it may be time for the practitioners to heal themselves and for administrators to consider that within short-term contexts of economic efficiency they are weaving the fabric of long-term distress in the nurses and doctors providing the service. Losing a sense of the sensual body, a sense of relationship and a spiritual understanding of dying is dangerous for all involved in the healing encounter: thus my repeated insistence that the delivery of medicine is more than its technologies.

If the progress of disease is an increasing personal isolation, then the therapeutic relationship is important for maintaining interpersonal contact. In this contact we are assisted in transcending the moment. In this transcendence, the essence of spirituality, we take a leap into a new consciousness of the vertical ecology, which is hope. That this new consciousness is not necessarily bound up with our bodies, our instincts, our motor impulses or our emotions awakens our awareness to another purpose within us. This awareness has implications for our bodies, our emotions, our awareness of others and our relationships. What I choose to call the horizontal ecology of our lives is a matter of belief for many of us. Demonstrating these material implications is the subject of a variety of work in psychoneuroimmunology (Kiecolt-Glaser and Glaser 1988, 1999), mind–body medicine (Dienstfrey 1992, 1999b; Lerner 1994) and spiritual healing (Benor 1992; Wirth 1993, 1995; Wirth and Cram 1997; Wirth *et al.* 1993, 1996a, 1996b).

In the face of no available cure, the practitioner is willing to consider comfort and relief as vital components of the therapy. Furthermore, the patient is often expected to play an active role in treatment. Something can be done. Not in the false hope of a cure, but in the true hope that it is possible to rise above the situation at hand. Optimism is making the best of the situation, even when the outcome is dire. Perhaps the psychological importance of hope is in the activity of hoping. It is not that a definite goal will be reached for the dying, but the possibility for transcendence. Such considerations are well within the range of conventional medicine, as palliative care has so ably demonstrated.

Yet there is also a vertical dimension to this ecology. We may all need at some time in our professional lives to face the questions of meaning and purpose, perhaps other than in crises of the clinical situation, which raises the issue of how we, the carers, care for each other. This may seem naive in a current health-care climate polluted by materialism and the notion of health as product. But surely we must pay heed to what our patients are demanding of us, even as they turn to practitioners of other persuasions than our own.

A vocabulary of healing

We have a long way to go yet in our understandings of the phenomena of what it means to be healed. My plea is simple – that we learn to accept and understand the expectations of our patients. Some authors have suggested that spiritual healing is the coming mode of medicine for this century. I would completely disagree. Clean water, adequate nutrition, protection from the vagaries of fire and flood, charity towards the poor and living in peace with our neighbours are, as in the past, of paramount importance for promoting and sustaining health in the world. To understand the symbolic meaning of these material realities and how we encourage their delivery is the challenge to medicine for this century. That these may be predicated upon a sacred understanding of human beings and nature that affects health-care delivery, which we may call spiritual, is vital.

It is important how we talk about healing and it is difficult to apply a spiritual vocabulary intelligibly because we are losing the use of certain terms. An understanding of grace, transcendence, forgiveness, reconciliation, redemption and sacrament are vital for accompanying our patients through the process of living, suffering and dying. Yet these words are strange to the vocabulary of both medical students and teachers. My call to the reader is not to abandon his or her vocabulary of science, but to enrich the vocabulary of healing even so far that we speak not only of *mind* and *body*, but also of *spirit*. In this way we transcend our normal existence to the very stuff of living. Words demand their usage to retain them within the culture. Furthermore, while *faith, hope, charity* and *love* may all be words that are in common usage, it would be a pity if we understood them only in their profane applications and abandoned their sacred dimensions.

Both medicine and spiritual healing can bring about the conditions in which healing can occur. But neither orthodox tradition, be it church or medicine, can explain how healing occurs. Nor will either until we begin to accept that our knowledge is wanting and our searching is misguided. Healing research or clinical outcome trials only measure the products or efficacy of healing endeavours. Our spiritual understanding of the intention of healing is lost. While we may know the social implications of healing such as integration into the community, improving and maintaining the available pool of labour, the psychological implications of healing such as happier, contented patients (Fehring, Brennan and Keller 1987) relieved of distress and sexually satisfied (Malatesta *et al.* 1988) and the physical implications of healing such as restored blood values, improved circulation and extended mobility, we remember little of the spiritual intentions of healing. Miracles had a deeper purpose other than the restoration of physical health. It is not that the age of miracles is past, rather that the spiritual understanding is hidden and has been supplanted by material and emotional satisfactions alone (Shah 1964).

The whole point of the spiritual argument, so aptly related in the Book of Job, is that the spirit leads we know not where. The generating of hypotheses restricts the changes to a range of possibilities, there is then no place for transcendence. As we have read in Chapter 6, no material change may occur in spiritual healing, but the individual transcends her immediate situation. Furthermore, there are no personal stories in medical science but group probabilities. This is seriously at odds with the demands of the patient's encounter with her doctor, which is personal. People are subjective, they are indeed subjects, and subjects that need to relate a story to another person who understands them. To be treated as objects in a world of social events deprives them of meaning. It is this very lack of meaning that exacerbates suffering.

Becoming sick, being treated, achieving recovery and becoming well are plots in the narrative of life. As such they are a reminder of our mortality. They are an historical relationship and meanings are linked together in time. Stories have a shape, they have purpose and are bounded in time. Thus, we talk about a case history. It is for this reason that group studies fail to offer an essential under-standing of what it is to fall ill and become well. Generalization loses individual intent and time is removed. The individual biographical historicity is lost in favour of the group. Purpose and intent are important in life, they are at the basis of hope. If that purpose is abandoned through hopelessness, then suicide and death are the outcome. In our healing endeavours we need to consider the circumstances in which healing occurs and how those circumstances are enabled. This is not the technological approach of cure but the ecological approach of providing the ground in which healing is achieved, whether it be an organic, psychological, social or spiritual context. Those healing contexts will also be part of a biography. They have an historicity and this must also be included. If this is acceptable for understanding such disparate processes as human immunity as it is for psychoanalysis, then there should be no major hindrance to understanding health as a developmental narrative.

At the heart of much scientific thinking in the medical world is a desire for prediction, to base treatment strategies and outcomes on a group statistic of probability. This is quite rightly explained as the desire to provide the optimum treatment and to eliminate false treatment that harms. Such a statement is also based upon belief, a touching faith in statistical reasoning. Behind this thinking is an assumption that tomorrow will be the same as today, that the future is predicated on the past.

What many patients want from their treatment, and the basis of their hope, is that tomorrow will not be the same as yesterday. It is understandable that practitioners want the security of providing the correct and appropriate treatment, but it also belies an underlying anxiety on their behalf about the circumstances of life. What if the future is not indeed predictable, that chance foils the noblest activities of us all or that there are purposes at play beyond the populations of our statistical reasoning? If religion was described as the opium of the people, then science has become its valium in its reluctance to face the anxiety of death. What we need to learn is to stand steadfast in the face of the anxiety that death causes as it echoes in our lives. That constant cycle of life and death, of which we are part, can be reconciled but not controlled. This is the message of all spiritual traditions and which health-care delivery has as its recurring, albeit hidden, theme.

Spirituality, religion and health

Spirituality lends meaning and purpose to our lives. These purposes help us transcend what we are. We are processes of individual development in relational contexts that are embedded within a cultural matrix. We are also developing understandings of truth, indeed, each one of us is an aspect of truth. These understandings are predicated on changes in consciousness achieved through transcending one state of consciousness to another. This dynamic process of transcendence is animated by forces or subtle energies. For some authors these energies are organized as information or energies that organize energies.

In terms of healing, spirituality encourages a change in consciousness such that the current situation can be transcended. How this is translated into concrete heath-care terms is problematic. For the worried, there is release from temporal concerns. For the anxious, there is comfort. For the dying, they see purpose. For those in pain, there is relief. For the chronically sick, there is hope. But when we look for concrete manifestations, they are elusive and not predictable at a level of straightforward correspondence. We are not going to see an immediate relief of suffering in all instances. My blood cell count may remain low, but my soul can fly. Am I healthy or not?

The definition of health faces the same dilemma as that of defining spirituality. While as health-care scientists we operationalize the concept of health, we may have to consider that when people are talking about falling ill and becoming well they are speaking of something called 'Health'. This process may not be linked as two ends of a bipolar construct. When we talk of health and illness, we may not necessarily be talking about the process of 'Health'.

Religions are developing to meet individual needs and alternative forms of celebration as Durkheim (1995) himself foresaw. Within these religions, as symbolic systems and repertoires of practices with their multiplicity of ever-changing texts, there will be individualized spiritualities. The same goes for health-care practices and the fluctuating definitions of health or Health and its symbols.

If each one of us is a living truth, then other truths are achieved through relationship as encounter. Through this encounter with a living universe, we expand into an ecology of knowledge. Science will be one way of structuring this encounter. Religion will offer us another. Spirituality establishes the encounter in both. This is the unity of consciousness, becoming whole and the basis of the healing endeavour. As each person progresses, wholeness is achieved at a different level of understanding. These understandings may be horizontal in a natural ecology, vertical in a divine ecology, or both. Spirituality enables the transcendence from one level to the next, incorporating new perspectives and reconciling contradictions. Thus we become whole as a person: realizing that our relationships have to be healed, we become reconciled as a community; realizing that there is strife and discord, we search for political accord; realizing that there is imbalance and a lack of harmony, we search for a reconciliation with nature; realizing that we are alone we reach out to the cosmos.

And then we return to the silence.

References

Albrecht, G. (1994) 'Subjective health assessment.' In C. Jenkinson (ed) *Measuring Health and Medical Outcomes.* London: UCL Press.

Aldridge, D. (1986) 'Licence to heal.' *Crucible,* April–June, 58–66.

Aldridge, D. (1987a) 'A community approach to cancer in families.' *Journal of Maternal and Child Health 12,* 182–185.

Aldridge, D. (1987b) 'Families, cancer and dying.' *Family Practice 4,* 212–218.

Aldridge, D. (1987c) *One Body: A Guide to Healing in the Church.* London: SPCK.

Aldridge, D. (1987d) 'A team approach to terminal care: Personal implications for patients and practitioners.' *Journal of the Royal College of General Practitioners 37,* 364.

Aldridge, D. (1988) 'Goal setting: The patient's assessment of outcome and recognition of therapeutic change.' *Complementary Medical Research 3,* 89–97.

Aldridge, D. (1990a) 'The delivery of health care alternatives.' *Journal of the Royal Society of Medicine 83,* 179–182.

Aldridge, D. (1990b) 'Making and taking health care decisions.' *Journal of the Royal Society of Medicine 83,* 720–723.

Aldridge, D. (1991a) 'Healing and medicine.' *Journal of the Royal Society of Medicine 84,* 516–518.

Aldridge, D. (1991b) 'Single case research designs for the clinician.' *Journal of the Royal Society of Medicine 84,* 249–252.

Aldridge, D. (1991c) 'Spirituality, healing and medicine.' *Journal of British General Practice 41,* 425–427.

Aldridge, D. (1992) 'The needs of individual patients in clinical research.' *Advances 8,* 4, 58–65.

Aldridge, D. (1994) 'Unconventional medicine in Europe.' *Advances 10,* 2, 52–60.

Aldridge, D. (1996) *Music Therapy Research and Practice in Medicine. From Out of the Silence.* London: Jessica Kingsley Publishers.

Aldridge, D. (1998) *Suicide: The Tragedy of Hopelessness.* London: Jessica Kingsley Publishers.

Aldridge, D. and Pietroni, P. (1987) 'Research trials in general practice: Towards a focus on clinical practice.' *Family Practice 4,* 311–315.

Aldridge, D. and Rossiter, J. (1983) 'A strategic approach to suicidal behaviour.' *Journal of Systemic and Strategic Therapies 2,* 4, 49–62.

Aldridge, D. and Rossiter, J. (1984) 'A strategic assessment of deliberate self harm.' *Journal of Family Therapy 6,* 119–132.

Aldridge, D. and Rossiter, J. (1985) 'Difficult patients, intractable symptoms and spontaneous recovery in suicidal behaviour.' *Journal of Systemic and Strategic Therapies 4,* 66–76.

Alter, J. (1996) 'Gandhi's body, Gandhi's truth. Nonviolence and the biomoral imperative of public health.' *Journal of Asian Studies 55,* 2, 301–322.

Alter, J. (1997) 'A therapy to live by: Public health, the self and nationalism in the practice of a North Indian yoga society.' *Medical Anthropology 17,* 309–335.

Andersen, J.Ø. (1995) *Lifestyles, Consumption and Alternative Therapies.* Troense: Odense University Press.

Angeletti, L., Agrimi, U., Curia, C., French, D. and Mariani-Constantini, R. (1992) 'Healing rituals and sacred serpents.' *The Lancet 340,* 223–225.

Aponte, H. (1998) 'Love, the spiritual wellspring of forgiveness: An example of spirituality in therapy.' *Journal of Family Therapy 20,* 1, 37–58.

Appleby, L. (1992) 'Suicide in psychiatric patients – risk and prevention.' *British Journal of Psychiatry 161*, 749–758.

Armstrong, D. (1995) 'The rise of surveillance medicine.' *Sociology of Health and Illness 17*, 3, 393–404.

Ashby, J. and Lenhart, R. (1994) 'Prayer as a coping strategy for chronic pain patients.' *Rehabilitation Psychology 39*, 3, 205–208.

Astin, J. (1997) 'Stress reduction through mindfulness meditation – effects on psychological symptomatology, sense of control, and spiritual experiences.' *Psychotherapy and Psychosomatics 66*, 2, 97–106.

Aylwin, S., Durand, S. and Wilson, K. (1985) 'Thinking symptoms and the common cold.' Psychology Society of Ireland Annual Conference Ennis, Ireland, November (personal communication).

Baker Eddy, M. (1971/1875) *Science and Health.* Boston: First Church of Christ Scientist.

Bartholome, W.G. (1996) 'Physician-assisted suicide, hospice, and rituals of withdrawal.' *Journal of Law of Medical Ethics 24*, 3, 233–236.

Baszanger, I. (1998) 'The work sites of an American interactionist: Anselm Strauss, 1917–1996.' *Symbolic Interaction 21*, 4, 353–378.

Bateson, G. (1972) *Steps to an Ecology of Mind.* New York: Ballantine.

Bateson, G. (1978) *Mind and Nature.* Glasgow: Fontana.

Bateson, G. (1991) *A Sacred Unity.* New York: HarperCollins.

Bearon, L. and Koenig, H. (1990) 'Religious cognitions and use of prayer in health and illness.' *Gerontologist 30*, 2, 249–253.

Beer, S. (1975) *Platform for Change.* London: Wiley.

Belcher, A., Dettmore, D. and Holzemer, S. (1989) 'Spirituality and sense of well-being in persons with AIDS.' *Holistic Nursing Practice 3*, 4, 16–25.

Benedikt, M. (1996) 'Complexity, value and the psychological postulates of economics.' *Critical Theory 10*, 4, 551–593.

Benor, D. (1990) 'Survey of spiritual healing.' *Complementary Medical Research 4*, 3, 9–33.

Benor, D. (1991) 'Spiritual healing in clinical practice.' *Nursing Times 87*, 44, 35–37.

Benor, D. (1992) *Healing Research*, vol. 1. München: Helix Editions.

Benson, H. (1993) 'The relaxation response.' In D. Goleman and J. Gurin (eds) *Mind Body Medicine.* New York: Consumer Reports Books, pp.233–257.

Berger, P. (1967) *The Sacred Canopy.* New York: Doubleday.

Bergmark, K. (1998) 'The Links and Alcoholics Anonymous: Two "AA" movements in Sweden.' In I. Eisenbach-Stagl and P. Rosenqvist (eds) *Diversity in Unity. Studies of Alcoholics Anonymous in Eight Societies.* Helsinki: Nordic Council for Alcohol and Drug Research, pp.75–89.

Biddle, S. (1995) 'Exercise and social health.' *Research Quarterly for Exercise and Sport 66*, 4, 292–297.

Bienenfeld, D., Koenig, H., Larson, D. and Sherrill, K. (1997) 'Psychosocial predictors of mental health in a population of elderly women – test of an explanatory model.' *American Journal of Geriatric Psychiatry 5*, 1, 43–53.

Bird-David, N. (1999) '"Animism" revisited: Personhood, environment, and relational epistemology.' *Current Anthropology 40*, S67–79.

Bloch, J. (1998) 'Alternative spirituality and environmentalism.' *Reviews of Religious Research 40*, 1, 55–73.

Blumer, H. (1972) 'Society as symbolic interaction.' In J. Manis and B. Metyler (eds) *Symbolic Interaction: A Reader in Social Psychology.* Boston: Allyn and Bacon.

Borman, P. and Dixon, D. (1998) 'Spirituality and the 12 steps of substance abuse recovery.' *Journal of Psychology and Theology 26*, 3, 287–291.

Bourdieu, P. (1993) *The Field of Cultural Production.* New York: Columbia University Press.

Bourjolly, J. (1998) 'Differences in religiousness among black and white women with breast cancer.' *Social Work in Health Care 28*, 1, 21–39.

Boutell, K. and Bozett, F. (1990) 'Nurses' assessment of patients' spirituality: Continuing education implications.' *Journal of Continuing Education in Nursing 21*, 4, 172–176.

Boyd, J. (1995) 'The soul as seen through evangelical eyes, part I: Mental health professionals and "the soul".' *Journal of Psychology and Theology 25*, 3, 151–160.

Brenner, M. (1987) 'Economic change, alcohol consumption and heart disease mortality in nine industrialized countries.' *Social Science and Medicine 25*, 2, 119–132.

Brewster Smith, M. (1994) 'Selfhood at risk: Postmodern perils and the perils of postmodernism.' *American Psychologist 49*, 5, 405–411.

Brown, C. (1995) 'Spiritual healing in general practice.' *Complementary Therapies in Medicine 3*, 230–233.

Brown, C. and Sheldon, M. (1989) 'Spiritual healing in general practice (letter).' *Journal of the Royal College of General Practitioners 39*, 328, 476–477.

Browner, C. (1998) 'Varieties of reasoning in medical anthropology.' *Medical Anthropology Quarterly 12*, 3, 356–362.

Bullis, R. (1991) The spiritual healing 'defense' in criminal prosecutions for crimes against children. *Child Welfare 70*, 5, 541–555.

Burkhardt, M. (1989) 'Spirituality: An analysis of the concept.' *Holistic Nursing Practitioner 3*, 3, 69–77.

Burkhardt, R. and Kienle, G. (1980) 'Controlled clinical trials and drug regulations.' *Controlled Clinical Trials 1*, 151–164.

Burkhardt, R. and Kienle, G. (1983) 'Basic problems in controlled trials.' *Journal of Medical Ethics 9*, 80–84.

Burkitt, I. (1998) 'Bodies of knowledge: Beyond Cartesian views of persons, selves and minds.' *Journal for the Theory of Social Behaviour 28*, 1, 63–82.

Burston, D. (1996) *The Wings of Madness: The Life and Work of R.D. Laing*. London: Harvard University Press.

Buxton, M., Smith, D. and Seymour, R. (1987) 'Spirituality and other points of resistance to the 12-step recovery process.' *Journal of Psychoactive Drugs 19*, 3, 275–286.

Byrd, R. (1988) 'Positive therapeutic effects of intercessory prayer in a coronary care unit population.' *Southern Medical Journal 81*, 7, 826–829.

Calhoun, B., Reitman, J. and Hoeldtke, N. (1997) 'Perinatal hospice: A response to partial birth abortion for infants with congenital defects.' *Issues, Law and Medicine 13*, 2, 125–143.

Campbell, C. (1998) 'Religion and the body in medical research.' *Kennedy Institute of Ethics Journal 8*, 3, 275–305.

Canale, J., White, R. and Kelly, K. (1996) 'The use of altruism and forgiveness in therapy.' *Journal of Religion and Health 35*, 3, 225–230.

Carey, G. (1997) 'Towards wholeness: Transcending the barriers between religion and psychiatry.' *British Journal of Psychiatry 170*, 396–397.

Carr, E. and Morris, T. (1996) 'Spirituality and patients with advanced cancer: A social work response.' *Journal of Psychosocial Oncology 14*, 1, 71–81.

Carroll, S. (1993) 'Spirituality and purpose in life in alcoholism recovery.' *Journal of Studies on Alcohol 54*, 3, 297–301.

Carson, V. and Green, H. (1992) 'Spiritual well-being: A predictor of hardiness in patients with acquired immunodeficiency syndrome.' *Journal of Professional Nursing 8*, 4, 209–220.

Cassell, E. (1991) *The Nature of Suffering and the Goals of Medicine*. New York: Oxford University Press.

Cavanaugh, M. (1994) 'The precursors of the Eureka moment as a common ground between science and theology.' *Zygon 29*, 2, 191–203.

Chandler, C., Holden, J. and Kolander, C. (1992) 'Counseling for spiritual wellness: Theory and practice.' *Journal of Counseling and Development 71*, 168–175.

Chang, B., Noonan, A. and Tennstedt, S. (1998) 'The role of religion/spirituality in coping with caregiving for disabled elders.' *Gerontologist 38*, 4, 463–470.

Charmaz, K. (1995) 'The body, identity, and self: Adapting to impairment.' *Sociological Quarterly 36*, 4, 657–680.

Chatters, L. and Taylor, R. (1989) 'Age differences in religious participation among black adults.' *Journal of Gerontology 44*, 5, S183–189.

Chatters, L., Levin, J. and Ellison, G. (1998) 'Public health and health education in faith communities.' *Health Education and Behavior 25*, 6, 869–899.

Clark, J. and Dawson, L. (1996) 'Personal religiousness and ethical judgements: An empirical analysis.' *Journal of Business Ethics 15*, 3, 359–372.

Clark, F., Carlson, M., Zemke, R., Frank, G., Patterson, K., Ennevor, B., Rankinmartinez, A., Hobson, L., Crandall, J., Mandel, D. and Lipson, L. (1996) 'Life domains and adaptive strategies of a group of low-income, well older adults.' *American Journal of Occupational Therapy 50*, 2, 99–108.

Cohen, J. (1989) 'Spiritual healing in a medical context.' *Practitioner 233*, 1473, 1056–1057.

Collipp, P. (1969) 'The efficacy of prayer: A triple blind study.' *Medical Times 97*, 201–204.

Compton, M. (1998) 'The union of religion and health in ancient Asklepieia.' *Journal of Religion and Health 37*, 4, 301–312.

Conrad, N. (1985) 'Spiritual support for the dying.' *Nursing Clinics of North America 20*, 2, 415–426.

Consoli, A. (1996) 'Psychotherapists' personal and mental health values according to their theoretical/professional orientation.' *Revista Interamericana de Psicologia 30*, 1, 59–83.

Conway, K. (1985) 'Coping with the stress of medical problems among black and white elderly.' *International Journal of Aging and Human Development 21*, 1, 39–48.

Cooke, M. (1992) 'Supporting health care workers in the treatment of HIV-infected patients.' *Primary Care 19*, 1, 245–256.

Courtenay, A. (1991) *Healing Now*. London: Dent.

Crombez, J.C. and Dubreuco, J.L. (1991) 'Can one die healed?' *Journal of Palliative Care 7*, 2, 39–43.

Crossley, N. (1995) 'Body techniques, agency and intercorporeality: On Goffman's relations in public.' *Sociology 29*, 1, 133–149.

Csordas, T. (1983) 'The rhetoric of transformation in ritual healing.' *Culture, Medicine and Psychiatry 7*, 4, 333–375.

Csordas, T. (1997) *The Sacred Self: A Cultural Phenomenology of Charismatic Healing*. Berkeley: University of California Press.

Cunningham, A. and Edmonds, C. (1996) 'Group psychological therapy for cancer patients: A point of view, and discussion of the hierarchy of options.' *International Journal of Psychiatry in Medicine 26*, 1, 51–82.

Cunningham, J., Sobell, L. and Sobell, M. (1996) 'Are diseases and other conceptions of alcohol abuse related to beliefs about outcomes?' *Journal of Applied Social Psychology 26*, 9, 773–780.

Cupitt, D. (1997) *After God. The Future of Religion*. New York: Basic Books.

Cutter, C. and Cutter, H. (1987) 'Experience and change in Al-Anon family groups: Adult children of alcoholics.' *Journal for the Study of Alcohol 48*, 1, 29–32.

Dallos, R. and Aldridge, D. (1986) 'Change: How do we recognise it?' *Journal of Family Therapy 8*, 45–59.

Davis, N.J. and Robinson, R.V. (1996) 'Are the rumors of war exaggerated? Religious orthodoxy and moral progressivism in America.' *American Jounral of Sociology 102*, 3, 756–787.

Dawson, L. (1998) 'The cultural significance of new religioused movements and globalization: A theoretical prolegomenon.' *Journal for the Scientific Study of Religion 37*, 4, 580–595.

Dawson, P.J. (1997) 'Spirituality as integrative energy – reply.' *Journal of Advance Nursing 25*, 2, 282–289.

Dienstfrey, H. (1992) 'Does spirit matter? Four perspectives.' *Advances 8*, 1, 31.

Dienstfrey, H. (1999a) 'Disclosure and health: An interview with James W. Pennebaker.' *Advances in Mind–Body Medicine 15*, 161–195.

Dienstfrey, H. (1999b) 'Mind and mindlessness in mind–body research.' *Advances in Mind–Body Medicine 15*, 229–233.

Dillon, K. and Baker, K. (1985) 'Positive emotional states and enhancement of the immune system.' *International Journal of Psychiatry 15*, 13–17.

Dillon, M.C. (1988) 'Mutumwa Nchimi healers and wizardry beliefs in Zambia.' *Social Science and Medicine 26*, 11, 1159–1172.

Dixon, M. (1998) 'Does "healing" benefit patients with chronic symptoms? A quasi-randomized trial in general practice.' *Journal of the Royal Society of Medicine 91*, 183–188.

Dohrenwend, B. and Dohrenwend, B. (1974) *Stressful Life Events: Their Nature and Effects.* New York: Wiley.

Dossey, B. (1999) 'Barbara Dossey on holistic nursing, Florence Nightingale, and healing rituals.' *Alternative Therapies 5*, 1, 79–86.

Dossey, L. (1982) *Space, Time and Medicine.* Boulder CO: Shambala.

Dossey, L. (1993) *Healing Words: The Power of Prayer and the Practice of Medicine.* New York: HarperCollins.

Downer, S., Cody, M., McCluskey, P., Wilson, P., Arnott, S., Lister, T. and Slevin, M. (1994) 'Pursuit and practice of complementary therapies by cancer patients receiving conventional treatment.' *British Medical Journal 309*, 86–89.

Doyle, D. (1992) 'Have we looked beyond the physical and psychosocial?' *Journal of Pain Symptom Management 7*, 5, 302–311.

Dreyfus, H. (1987) 'Foucault's critique of psychiatric medicine.' *Journal of Medicine and Philosophy 12*, 311–333.

Duckro, P. and Magaletta, P. (1994) 'The effect of prayer on physical health: Experimental evidence.' *Journal of Religion and Health 33*, 3, 211–219.

Dull, V. and Skokan, L. (1995) 'A cognitive model of religion's influence on health.' *Journal of Social Issues 51*, 2, 49–64.

Durkheim, E. (1958) *The Rules of Sociological Method.* Trans. S.A. Soloray and J.H. Mueller. New York: Free Press.

Durkheim, E. (1995) *The Elementary Forms of Religious Life.* New York: Free Press.

Duvall, N. (1998) 'From soul to self and back again.' *Journal of Psychology and Theology 26*, 1, 6–15.

Eisenbach-Stagl, I. (1998) 'How to live a sober life in a wet society: Alcoholics Anonymous in Austria.' In I. Eisenbach-Stagl and P. Rosenqvist (eds) *Diversity in Unity. Studies of Alcoholics Anonymous in Eight Societies.* Helsinki: Nordic Council for Alcohol and Drug Research, pp.131–147.

Eisenberg, L. (1992) 'Treating depression and anxiety in primary care. Closing the gap between knowledge and practice.' *New England Journal of Medicine 326*, 16, 1080–1084.

Eliade, M. (1989) *Shamanism: Archaic Techniques of Ecstasy.* London: Arkana.

Elias, P. (1996) 'Worklessness and social pathologies in Aboriginal communities.' *Human Organization 55*, 1, 13–24.

Emblen, J. (1992) 'Religion and spirituality defined according to current use in nursing literature.' *Journal of Professional Nursing 8*, 1, 41–47.

Engebretson, J. (1996) 'Urban healers: An experiential description of American healing touch groups.' *Qualitative Health Research 6*, 4, 526–541.

Erikson, K. (1966) *Wayward Puritans.* New York: Wiley.

Estes, J.W. (1991) 'The Shakers and their proprietary medicines.' *Bulletin of Historical Medicine 65*, 2, 162–184.

Evans, G., Barer, M. and Marmor, T. (1994) *Why Are Some People Healthy and Others Not?* New York: Aldine de Gruyter.

Fabrega, H. (1997) 'Earliest phases in the evolution of sickness and healing.' *Medical Anthropology Quarterly 11*, 1, 26–55.

Farquhar, J. (1994) 'Eating Chinese medicine.' *Cultural Anthropology 9*, 4, 471–497.

Fehring, R., Brennan, P. and Keller, M. (1987) 'Psychological and spiritual well-being in college students.' *Research in Nursing and Health 10*, 6, 391–398.

Ferch, S. (1998) 'Intentional forgiving as a counseling intervention.' *Journal of Counseling Development 76*, 3, 261–270.

Ferrell, B., Grant, M., Funk, B., OtisGreen, S. and Garcia, N. (1998) 'Quality of life in breast cancer part II: Psychological and spiritual well-being.' *Cancer Nursing 21*, 1, 1–9.

Finkler, K. (1994) 'Sacred healing and biomedicine compared.' *Medical Anthropology Quarterly 8*, 2, 178–197.

Fischer, S. and Johnson, P. (1999) 'Therapeutic touch: A viable link in midwifery.' *Journal of Nurse-Midwifery 44*, 3, 300–309.

Flaskerud, J. and Rush, C. (1989) 'AIDS and traditional health beliefs and practices of black women.' *Nursing Research 38*, 4, 210–215.

Foley, L., Wagner, J. and Waskel, S. (1998) 'Spirituality in the lives of older women.' *Journal of Women and Aging 10*, 2, 85–91.

Folkins, C. (1970) 'Temporal factors and the cognitive mediators of stress reaction.' *Journal of Personality and Social Psychology 14*, 173–184.

Ford, G. (1996) 'An existential model for promoting life change.' *Journal of Substance Abuse Treatment 13*, 2, 151–158.

Foucault, M. (1985) *The Use of Pleasure: The History of Sexuality Volume 2*. Harmondsworth: Penguin.

Foucault, M. (1989) *The Birth of the Clinic*. London: Routledge.

Frances, R. and Borg, L. (1993) 'The treatment of anxiety in patients with alcoholism.' *Journal of Clinical Psychiatry 54*, supplement, 37–43.

Fransella, F. and Frost, K. (1977) *On Being a Woman: A Review of Research on how Women See Themselves*. London: Tavistock.

Frohock, F. (1993) *Healing Powers*. Chicago: University of Chicago Press.

Furnham, A. and Boughton, J. (1995) 'Eating behaviour and body dissatisfaction among dieters, aerobic exercisers and a control group.' *European Eating Disorders Review 3*, 1, 35–45.

Furnham, A., Titman, P. and Sleeman, E. (1994) 'Perception of female body shapes as a function of exercise.' *Journal of Social Behavior and Personality 9*, 2, 335–352.

Ganz, P. (1992) 'Treatment options for breast cancer – beyond survival.' *New England Journal of Medicine 326*, 1147–1149.

Ganzevoort, R. (1998) 'Religious coping considered, part one: An integrated approach.' *Journal of Psychology and Theology 26*, 3, 260–275.

Garrett, G. (1991) 'A natural way to go? Death and bereavement in old age.' *Professional Nurse 6*, 12, 744–746.

Geertz, C. (1957) 'Ritual and social change.' *American Anthropologist 59*, 32–54.

Gergen, K. (1991) *The Saturated Self: Dilemmas of Identity in Contemporary Life*. New York: Basic Books.

Gergen, K. (1997) 'Psycho- versus bio-medical therapy.' *Society 35*, 1, 24–27.

Gillespie, M. (1998) 'Nietzsche and the premodernist critique of postmodernity.' *Critical Review 11*, 4, 537–554.

Glik, D. (1988) 'Symbolic, ritual and social dynamics of spiritual healing.' *Social Science and Medicine 27*, 11, 1197–1206.

Gold, R. (1995) 'Why we need to rethink AIDS education for gay men.' *AIDS Care 7*, supplement 1, S11–19.

Goleman, D. and Gurin, J. (1993) *Mind Body Medicine*. New York: Consumer Reports Books.

Gorham, M. (1989) 'Spirituality and problem solving with seniors.' *Perspectives 13*, 3, 13–16.

Grad, B., Cadoret, R. and Paul, G. (1961) 'The influence of an unorthodox method of treatment on wound healing in mice.' *International Journal of Parapsychology 3*, 5–24.

Grasser, C. and Craft, B. (1984) 'The patient's approach to wellness.' *Nursing Clinics of North America 19*, 2, 207–218.

Greco, M. (1998a) 'Between social and organic norms: Reading Canguilhem and "somatization".' *Economy and Society 27*, 2/3, 234–248.

Greco, M. (1998b) 'The time of the real: When disease is "actual".' *Cultural Values 2*, 2/3, 243–260.

Green, L., Fullilove, M. and Fullilove, R. (1998) 'Stories of spiritual awakening – the nature of spirituality in recovery.' *Journal of Substance Abuse Treatment 15*, 4, 325–331.

Greisinger, A., Lorimor, R., Aday, L., Winn, R. and Baile, W. (1997) 'Terminally ill cancer patients – their most important concerns.' *Cancer Practice 5*, 3, 147–154.

Griffith, E. (1983) 'The significance of ritual in a church-based healing model.' *American Journal of Psychiatry 140*, 5, 568–572.

Griffith, E. and Mahy, G. (1984) 'Psychological benefits of Spiritual Baptist "mourning".' *American Journal of Psychiatry 141*, 6, 769–773.

Griffith, E., Mahy, G. and Young, J. (1986) 'Psychological benefits of Spiritual Baptist "mourning," II: An empirical assessment.' *American Journal of Psychiatry 143*, 2, 226–229.

Grivetti, L., Lamprecht, S., Rocke, H. and Waterman, A. (1987) 'Threads of cultural nutrition: arts and humanities.' *Progress in Food and Nutrition Science 11*, 3/4, 249–306.

Gutterman, L. (1990) 'A day treatment program for persons with AIDS.' *American Journal of Occupational Therapy 44*, 3, 234–237.

Hagelin, J., Rainforth, M., Orme-Johnson, D., Cavanaugh, K., Alexander, C., Shatkin, S., Davies, J., Hughes, A. and Ross, E. (1999) 'Effects of group practice of the transcendental meditation program on preventing violent crime in Washington, D.C.: Results of the national demonstration project, June–July 1993.' *Social Indicators Research 47*, 153–201.

Haley, J. (1980) *Leaving Home.* New York: McGraw-Hill.

Hall, B. (1998) 'Patterns of spirituality in persons with advanced HIV disease.' *Research in Nursing and Health 21*, 143–153.

Hamilton, M., Waddington, P., Gregory, S. and Walker, A. (1995) 'Eat, drink and be saved: The spiritual significance of alternative diets.' *Social Compass 42*, 4, 497–511.

Hanegraaff, W. (1999) 'New Age spiritualities as secular religion: A historian's perspective.' *Social Compass 46*, 2, 145–160.

Hansen, D. and Hill, R. (1964) 'Families under stress.' In H. Christensen (ed) *Handbook of Marriage and the Family.* Chicago: Rand McNally.

Hansen, D. and Johnson, V. (1979) 'Rethinking family stress theory: Definitional aspects.' In W. Burr, R. Hill, F. Nye and D. Reiss (eds) *Contemporary Theories about the Family.* New York: Free Press, pp.582–603.

Hargrave, T. and Sells, J. (1997) 'The development of a forgiveness scale.' *Journal of Marital and Family Therapy 23*, 1, 41–63.

Harrington, V., Lackey, N. and Gates, M. (1996) 'Needs of caregivers of clinic and hospice cancer patients.' *Cancer Nursing 19*, 2, 118–125.

Hawton, K., Fagg, J., Platt, S. and Hawkins, M. (1993) 'Factors associated with suicide after parasuicide in young people.' *British Medical Journal 306*, 6893, 1641–1644.

Hay, D. and Morisy, A. (1985) 'Secular society, religious meanings: A contemporary paradox.' *Reviews of Religious Research 26*, 3, 213–227.

Heidegren, C. (1997) 'Transcendental theory of society, anthropology and the sociology of law: Helmut Schelsky – an almost forgotten sociologist.' *Acta Sociologica 40*, 3, 279–290.

Helman, C. (1984) *Culture, Health and Illness.* Bristol: Wright.

Helman, C. (1986) 'The consultation in context.' *Holistic Medicine 1*, 37–41.

Henriksson, M., Aro, H., Marttunen, M., Heikkinen, M., Isometsa, E., Kuoppasalmi, K. and Lonnqvist, J. (1993) 'Mental disorders and comorbidity in suicide.' *American Journal of Psychiatry 150*, 6, 935–940.

Hiatt, J. (1986) 'Spirituality, medicine, and healing.' *Southern Medical Journal 79*, 6, 736–743.

Higginson, I., Wade, A. and McCarthy, K. (1992) 'Effectiveness of two palliative support teams.' *Journal of Public Health Medicine 14*, 1, 50–56.

Highfield, M. (1992) 'Spiritual health of oncology patients. Nurse and patient perspectives.' *Cancer Nursing 15*, 1, 1–8.

Hileman, J., Lackey, N. and Hassanein, R. (1992) 'Identifying the needs of home caregivers of patients with cancer.' *Oncology Nursing Forum 19*, 5, 771–777.

Hoffman, L. (1985) 'Beyond power and control: Toward a "second order" family systems therapy.' *Family Systems Medicine 3*, 381–396.

Holt, J., Houg, B. and Romano, J. (1999) 'Spiritual wellness for clients with HIV/AIDS: Review of counselling issues.' *Journal of Counselling and Development 77*, 160–170.

Hossein Nasr, S. (1990) *Man and Nature: The Spiritual Crisis in Modern Man.* London: Unwin.

Hunt, S. (1985) 'Measuring health status: A new tool for clinicians and epidemiologists.' *Journal of the Royal College of General Practitioners 35*, 185–188.

Idinopulos, T. (1998) 'What is religion?' *Cross Currents 48*, 3, 366–380.

Idler, E. (1995) 'Religion, health and the nonphysical senses of self.' *Social Forces 74*, 22, 683–704.

Idler, E. and Kasl, S. (1997) 'Religion among disabled and nondisabled persons. 1. Cross-sectional patterns in health practices, social activities, and well-being.' *Journals of Gerontology Series B – Psychological Sciences and Social Sciences 52*, 6, S294–S305.

Inglis, B. (1979) *Natural Medicine*. Glasgow: Fontana Collins.

Irving, L., Snyder, C. and Crowson, J. (1998) 'Hope and coping with cancer by college women.' *Journal of Personality 66*, 2, 195–214.

Jackson, D. (1965) 'Family rules: Marital quid pro quo.' *Archives of General Psychiatry 12*, 589–594.

Jacobs, S. (1989) 'A philosophy of energy.' *Holistic Medicine 4*, 95–111.

Jenkins, R.A. (1995) 'Religion and HIV: Implications for research and intervention.' *Journal of Social Issues 51*, 2, 131–144.

Joseph, M. (1998) 'The effect of strong religious beliefs on coping with stress.' *Stress Medicine 14*, 219–224.

Joyce, C. and Welldon, R. (1965) 'The efficacy of prayer: A double-blind clinical trial.' *Journal of Chronic Diseases 18*, 367–377.

Jung, C. (1961) *Modern Man in Search of a Soul*. London: Routledge and Kegan Paul.

Kabat-Zinn, J. (1993) 'Mindfulness meditation: Health benefits of an ancient Buddhist practice.' In D. Goleman and J. Gurin (eds) *Mind Body Medicine*. New York: Consumer Reports Books, pp.259–275.

Kaczorowski, J. (1989) 'Spiritual well-being and anxiety in adults diagnosed with cancer.' *Hospital Journal 5*, 3/4, 105–116.

Kaplan, M., Marks, G. and Mertens, S. (1997) 'Distress and coping among women with HIV infection: Preliminary findings from a multiethnic sample.' *American Journal of Orthopsychiatry 67*, 1, 80–91.

Kelly, M. and Field, D. (1996) 'Medical sociology, chronic illness and the body.' *Sociology of Health and Illness 18*, 2, 241–257.

Kendler, K.S., Gardner, C.O. and Prescott, C.A. (1997) 'Religion, psychopathology, and substance use and abuse: A multimeasure, genetic-epidemiologic study.' *American Journal of Psychiatry 154*, 3, 322–329.

Khan, I. (1974) *The Development of Spiritual Healing*. Claremont CA: Hunter House.

Khan, I. (1979) *The Bowl of Saki*. Geneva: Sufi Publishing.

Khan, I. (1983) *The Music of Life*. Santa Fe: Omega Press.

Kiecolt-Glaser, J. and Glaser, R. (1988) 'Psychological influences on immunity.' *American Psychologist 43*, 11, 892–898.

Kiecolt-Glaser, J. and Glaser, R. (1999) 'Psychoneuroimmunology and immunotoxicology: Implications for carcinogenesis.' *Psychosomatic Medicine 61*, 271–272.

Kiecolt-Glaser, J., Cacioppo, J., Malarkey, W. and Glaser, R. (1992) 'Acute psychological stressors and short-term immune changes – what, why, for whom, and to what extent?' *Psychosomatic Medicine 54*, 6, 680–685.

King, D., Sobal, J., Haggerty, J., Dent, M. and Patton, D. (1992) 'Experiences and attitudes about faith healing among family physicians.' *Journal of Family Practice 35*, 2, 158–162.

King, M.B. (1997) 'Psychiatry and religion, context, consensus and controversies, by D. Bhugra.' *British Journal of Psychiatry 170*, 93–94.

King, M. and Dein, S. (1998) 'The spiritual variable in psychiatric research.' *Psychological Medicine 28*, 1259–1262.

King, M., Speck, P. and Thomas, A. (1994) 'Spiritual and religious beliefs in acute illness – is this a feasible area for study?' *Social Science in Medicine 38*, 4, 631–636.

King, M., Speck, P. and Thomas, A. (1995) 'The Royal Free interview for religious and spiritual beliefs: Devleopment and standardization.' *Psychological Medicine 25*, 1125–1134.

King, M., Speck, P. and Thomas, A. (1999) 'The effect of spiritual outcome from illness.' *Social Science and Medicine 48*, 1291–1299.

Kirkwood, W. and Brown, D. (1995) 'Public communication about the causes of disease: The rhetoric of responsibility.' *Journal of Communication 45*, 1, 55–76.

Kirmayer, L. (1993) 'Healing and the intervention of metaphor.' *Culture, Medicine and Psychiatry 17*, 161–195.

Kleinman, A. (1973) 'Medicine's symbolic reality. On a central problem in the philosophy of medicine.' *Inquiry 16*, 206–213.

Kleinman, A. (1978) 'Culture, illness and care.' *Annals of Internal Medicine 88*, 251–258.

Kleinman, A. (1980) *Patients and Healers in the Context of Culture.* Berkeley: University of California Press.

Kleinman, A. and Sung, L. (1979) 'Why do indigenous practitioners successfully heal?' *Social Science and Medicine 13*, 7–26.

Klingbeil, B. (1993) *The Spindrift Papers: Exploring Prayer and Healing through the Experimental Test. Volume I 1975–1993.* Lansdale PA: Spindrift.

Klivington, K. (1997) 'Information, energy, and healing: Challenges to biology and medicine.' *Advances 13*, 4, 3–6, 36–42.

Koenig, H., Bearon, L. and Dayringer, R. (1989) 'Physician perspectives on the role of religion in the physician, older patient relationship.' *Journal of Family Practice 28*, 4, 441–448.

Koenig, H., Hays, J., George, L., Blazer, D., Larson, D. and Landerman, L. (1997) 'Modeling the cross-sectional relationships between religion, physical health, social support, and depressive symptoms.' *American Journal of Geriatric Psychiatry 5*, 2, 131–144.

Koenig, H., George, L. and Peterson, B. (1998a) 'Religiosity and remission of depression in medically ill older patients.' *American Journal of Psychiatry 155*, 4, 536–542.

Koenig, H., Pargament, K. and Nielsen, J. (1998b) 'Religious coping and health status in medically ill hospitalized older adults.' *Journal of Nervous and Mental Disease 186*, 9, 513–521.

Krause, N. (1998) 'Neighborhood deterioration, religious coping and changes in health during late life.' *Gerontological Society of America 38*, 6, 653–664.

Kreitman, N., Smith, P. and Eng-Seong, T. (1969) 'Attempted suicide in social networks.' *British Journal of Preventive Social Medicine 23*, 116–123.

Krieger, D. (1979) *The Therapeutic Touch.* Englewood Cliffs: Prentice Hall.

Kurtz, E. (1979) *Not-God. A History of Alcoholics Anonymous.* Center City MN: Hazelden Pittman Archives Press.

Labun, E. (1988) 'Spiritual care: An element in nursing care planning.' *Journal of Advanced Nursing 13*, 3, 314–320.

Lapierre, L. (1994) 'A model for describing spirituality.' *Journal of Religion and Health 33*, 2, 153–161.

Larner, G. (1998) 'Through a glass darkly.' *Theory and Psychology 8*, 4, 549–572.

Lawton, J. (1998) 'Contemporary hospice care: The sequestration of the unbounded body and "dirty dying".' *Sociology of Health and Illness 20*, 2, 121–143.

Lazarus, R. (1974) 'Psychological stress and coping in adaptation and illness.' *International Journal of Psychiatry in Medicine 5*, 321–333.

Leach, E. (1976) *Culture and Communication: The Logic by which Symbols are Connected.* London: Cambridge University Press.

Lepine, J., Chignon, J. and Teherani, M. (1993) 'Suicide attempts in patients with panic disorder.' *Archives of General Psychiatry 50*, 2, 144–149.

Lerner, M. (1994) *Choices in Healing.* London: MIT Press.

Leskowitz, E. (1992) 'Life energy and western medicine: A reappraisal.' *Advances 8*, 1, 63–67.

Levin, J. and Schiller, P. (1987) 'Is there a religious factor in health?' *Journal of Religion and Health 26*, 1, 9–36.

Lewis-Fernandez, R. and Kleinman, A. (1994) 'Culture, personality and psychopathology.' *Journal of Abnormal Psychology 103*, 1, 67–71.

Lewith, G. and Aldridge, D. (1991) *Complementary Medicine and the European Community.* Saffron Walden: C.W. Daniel.

Liebermann, S. (1995) 'Anorexia nervosa: The tyranny of appearances.' *Journal of Family Therapy 17*, 1, 133–138.

Long, A. (1997) 'Nursing: A spiritual perspective.' *Nurse Ethics 4*, 6, 496–510.

Loudou, J. and Frankenberg, R. (1976) 'Social anthropology and medicine.' *ASAC Monograph 13*, 223–258.

Lowell Lewis, J. (1995) 'Genre and embodiment: From Brazilian Capoeira to the ethnology of human movement.' *Cultural Anthropology 10*, 2, 221–243.

Lukoff, D., Lu, F. and Turner, R. (1998) 'From spiritual emergency to spiritual problem: The transpersonal roots of the new DSM-IV category.' *Journal of Humanistic Psychology 38*, 2, 21–50.

Lukoff, D., Provenzano, R., Lu, F. and Turner, R. (1999) 'Religious and spiritual case reports on medline: A systematic analysis of records from 1980 to 1996.' *Alternative Therapies 5*, 1, 64–70.

Lynch, P. (1995) 'Adolescent smoking – an alternative perspective using personal construct theory.' *Health Education Research 10*, 1, 187–198.

McCarthy, K. (1984) 'Early alcoholism treatment: The Emmanuel Movement and Richard Peabody.' *Journal for the Study of Alcohol 45*, 1, 59–74.

McCullough, M. (1995) 'Prayer and health: Conceptual issues, research view, and research agenda.' *Journal of Psychology and Theology 25*, 1, 15–29.

McGuire, M. (1988) *Ritual Healing in Suburban America*. New Brunswik, NJ: Rutgers University Press.

McGuire, M. (1996) 'Religion and healing the mind/body/self.' *Social Compass 43*, 1, 101–116.

McKinney, J. and McKinney, K. (1999) 'Prayer in the lives of late adolescents.' *Journal of Adolescence 22*, 279–290.

McMillan, S. and Weitzner, M. (1998) 'Quality of life in cancer patients – use of a revised hospice index.' *Cancer Practice 6*, 5, 282–288.

McSherry, W. and Draper, P. (1997) 'The spiritual dimension: Why the absence within the nursing curricula?' *Nurse Education Today 17*, 413–417.

Madanes, C. (1981) *Strategic Family Therapy*. San Francisco: Jossey-Bass.

Magaletta, P. and Brawer, P. (1996) 'The use of prayer in psychotherapy: Ethical considerations (personal communication).' Paper presented at the American Psychological Association Annual Meeting, Toronto, 11 August.

Magaletta, P. and Brawer, P. (1998) 'Prayer in psychotherapy. A model for its use, ethical considerations, and guidelines for practice.' *Journal of Psychology and Theology 26*, 4, 322–330.

Magaletta, P. and Duckro, P. (1996) 'Prayer in the medical encounter.' *Journal of Religion and Health 35*, 3, 203–209.

Malatesta, V., Chambless, D., Pollack, M. and Cantor, A. (1988) 'Widowhood, sexuality and aging: A life span analysis.' *Journal of Sexual and Marital Therapy 14*, 1, 49–62.

Malson, H. (1999) 'Women under erasure. Anorexic bodies in postmodern context.' *Journal of Community and Applied Social Psychology 9*, 137–153.

Markides, K. (1983) 'Aging, religiosity, and adjustment: A longitudinal analysis.' *Journal of Gerontology 38*, 5, 621–625.

Markova, I. (1997) 'Language and authenticity.' *Journal for the Theory of Social Behaviour 27*, 2, 265–275.

Markush, R. (1974) 'Mental epidemics – a review of the old to prepare for the new.' *Public Health Reviews 11*, 4, 353–442.

Marsham, R. (1990) 'Sufi orders.' In I. Shah (ed) *Sufi Thought and Action*. London: Octagon Press, pp.112–122.

Martinez III, T. (1998) 'Anthropos and existence: Gnostic parallels in the early writings of Rollo May.' *Journal of Humanistic Psychology 38*, 4, 95–109.

Marx, K. (1964) *Early Writings*. New York: McGraw-Hill.

Mathew, R., Georgi, J., Wilson, W. and Mathew, V. (1996) 'A retrospective study of the concept of spirituality as understood by recovering individuals.' *Journal of Substance Abuse Treatment 13*, 1, 67–73.

May, C. (1997) 'Habitual drunkards and the invention of alcoholism: Susceptibility and culpability in nineteenth century medicine.' *Addiction Research 5*, 2, 169–187.

May, L. (1995) 'Challenging medical authority: The refusal of treatment by Christian Scientists.' *Hastings Center Report 25*, 1, 15–21.

Mechanic, D. (1966) 'Response factors in illness: The study of illness behaviour.' *Social Psychiatry 1*, 11–20.

Mechanic, D. (1974) 'Social structure and personal adaptation: Some neglected dimensions.' In G. Coelho, D. Hamburg and J. Adams (eds) *Coping and Adaptation*. New York: Basic Books.

Mehta, S. and Farina, A. (1997) 'Is being "sick" really better? Effect of the disease view of mental disorder on stigma.' *Journal of Social and Clinical Psychology 16*, 4, 405–419.

Meillier, L., Lund, A. and Kok, G. (1996) 'Reactions to health education among men.' *Health Education Research 11*, 1, 107–115.

Merleau-Ponty, M. (1962) *The Phenomenology of Perception.* London: Routledge and Kegan Paul.

Mermann, A. (1992) 'Spiritual aspects of death and dying.' *Yale Journal of Biological Medicine 65*, 2, 137–142.

Merrick, J. (1994) 'Christian Science healing of minor children: Spiritual exemption statutes, first amendment rights and fair notice.' *Issues in Law and Medicine 10*, 3, 321–342.

Merton, T. (1996) *A Search for Solitude: Pursuing the Monk's True Life.* In L. Cunningham (ed). New York: HarperCollins.

Merton, T. (1998) *The Other Side of the Mountain: The End of the Journey.* In P. Hart (ed). New York: HarperCollins.

Miller, L. and Finnerty, M. (1996) 'Sexuality, pregnancy, and childrearing among women with schizophrenia-spectrum disorders.' *Psychiatric Services 47*, 5, 502–506.

Miller, R. (1998a) 'Epistemology and psychotherapy data: The unspeakable, unbearable, horrible truth.' *Clinical Psychology: Science and Practice 5*, 2, 242–250.

Miller, W. (1998b) 'Researching the spiritual dimensions of alcohol and other drug problems.' *Addiction 93*, 7, 979–990.

Minuchin, S. (1974) *Families and Family Therapy.* Cambridge MA: Harvard University Press.

Minuchin, S., Baker, L., Rosman, B., Liebman, R., Milman, L. and Todd, T. (1975) 'A conceptual model of psychosomatic illness in children.' *Archives of General Psychiatry 32*, 1031–1038.

Moerman, D. (1998) 'Medical romanticism and the sources of medical practice.' *Complementary Therapies in Medicine 6*, 4, 198–202.

Montelpare, W. and Kanters, M. (1994) 'Symptom reporting, perceived health and leisure pursuits.' *Health Values 18*, 5, 34–40.

Musick, M., Koenig, H., Hays, J. and Cohen, H. (1998) 'Religious activity and depression among community-dwelling elderly persons with cancer: The moderating effect of race.' *Journals of Gerontology Series B – Psychological Sciences and Social Sciences 53*, 4, S218–S227.

Nagai Jacobson, M. and Burkhardt, M. (1989) 'Spirituality: Cornerstone of holistic nursing practice.' *Holistic Nursing Practitioner 3*, 3, 18–26.

Navarro, J., Wilson, S., Berger, L. and Taylor, T. (1997) 'Substance abuse and spirituality: A program for native American students.' *American Journal of Health Behavior 21*, 1, 3–11.

Needleman, J. (1988) *A Sense of the Cosmos.* London: Arkana.

NFSH (1999) *National Federation of Spiritual Healers Code of Conduct.* Sunbury on Thames: NFSH.

Nguyen, M., Otis, J. and Potvin, L. (1996) 'Determinants of intention to adopt a low-fat diet in men 30 to 60 years old: Implications for health promotion.' *American Journal of Health Promotion 10*, 3, 201–207.

Nicosia, G. (1983) *Memory Babe: A Critical Biography of Jack Kerouac.* Berkeley: University of California Press.

Nixon, P., Al Abbasi, A., King, J. and Freeman, L. (1986) 'Hyperventilation in cardiac rehabilitation.' *Holistic Medicine 1*, 5–13.

Orr, R. and Genesen, L. (1998) 'Medicine, ethics and religion: Rational or irrational.' *Journal of Medical Ethics 24*, 385–387.

Palmer, M. (1996) *The Book of Chang Tzu.* London: Arkana.

Pargament, K. and Park, C. (1995) 'Merely a defense? The variety of religious means and ends.' *Journal of Social Issues 51*, 2, 13–32.

Park, K. (1998) 'The religious construction of sanctuary provision in two congregations.' *Sociological Spectrum 18*, 393–421.

Parker, P. (1997) 'Suffering, prayer, and miracles.' *Journal of Religion and Health 36*, 3, 205–219.

Parsons, T. (1951) *The Social System.* New York: Free Press.

Pennebaker, J., Kiecolt-Glaser, J. and Glaser, R. (1988) 'Disclosure of traumas and immune function: Health implications for psychotherapy.' *Journal of Consulting and Clinical Psychology 56*, 239–245.

Perrett, R.W. (1996) 'Buddhism, euthanasia and the sanctity of life.' *Journal of Medical Ethics 22*, 5, 309–313.

Peteet, J. (1993) 'A closer look at the role of a spiritual approach in addictions treatment.' *Journal of Substance Abuse Treatment 10*, 3, 263–267.

Peteet, J., Stomper, P., Ross, D., Cotton, V., Truesdell, P. and Moczynski, W. (1992) 'Emotional support for patients with cancer who are undergoing CT: Semistructured interviews of patients at a cancer institute.' *Radiology 182*, 1, 99–102.

Pietroni, P.C. (1986) 'Spiritual interventions in a general practice setting.' *Holistic Medicine 1*, 253–262.

Pingleton, J. (1997) 'Why we don't forgive: A biblical and object relations theoretical model for understanding failures in the forgiveness process.' *Journal of Psychology and Theology 25*, 4, 403–413.

Pollard, M., Anderson, R., Anderson, W. and Jennings, G. (1998) 'The development of a family forgiveness scale.' *Journal of Family Therapy 20*, 1, 95–109.

Potts, R. (1996) 'Spirituality and the experience of cancer in an African-American community: Implications for psychosocial oncology.' *Journal of Psychosocial Oncology 14*, 1, 1–19.

Rawls, A. (1996a) 'Durkheim's epistemology: The initial critique, 1915–1924.' *Sociological Quarterly 38*, 1, 111–145.

Rawls, A. (1996b) 'Durkheim's epistemology: The neglected argument.' *American Journal of Sociology 102*, 2, 430–482.

Reason, P. and Rowan, J. (1981) *Human Inquiry*. Chichester: Wiley.

Reed, P. (1987) 'Spirituality and well-being in terminally ill hospitalized adults.' *Research in Nursing and Health 10*, 5, 335–344.

Reese, H. (1997) 'Spirituality, belief, and action.' *Journal of Mind and Behavior 18*, 1, 29–51.

Reiss, D. (1981) *The Family's Construction of Reality*. Cambridge MA: Harvard University Press.

Reiss, D. and Oloveri, M. (1983) 'Family stress as community frame.' *Marriage and Family Review 6*, 61–83.

Ribble, D. (1989) 'Psychosocial support groups for people with HIV infection and AIDS.' *Holistic Nursing Practice 3*, 4, 52–62.

Richards, T. and Folkman, S. (1997) 'Spiritual aspects of loss at the time of a partner's death from AIDS.' *Death Studies 21*, 6, 527–552.

Riis, O. (1998) 'Religion re-emerging. The role of religion in legitimating integration and power in modern societies.' *International Sociology 13*, 2, 249–272.

Roche, J. (1989) 'Spirituality and the ALS patient.' *Rehabilitation Nurse 14*, 3, 139–141.

Rodriguez, J. (1999) 'Towards an understanding of spirituality in U.S. Latina leadership.' *Frontiers – A Journal of Women Studies 20*, 1, 137–146.

Roof, W. (1998) 'Modernity, the religious, and the spiritual.' *Annals of the American Academy of Psychology, Society and Spirituality 558*, 211–224.

Rosner, F. (1975) 'The efficacy of prayer: Scientific v. religious evidence.' *Journal of Religion and Health 14*, 294–298.

Ross, L. (1994) 'Spiritual aspects of nursing.' *Journal of Advanced Nursing 19*, 439–447.

Ross, L. (1995) 'The spiritual dimension: Its importance to patients' health, well-being and quality of life and its implications for nursing practice.' *International Journal of Nurse Studies 32*, 5, 457–468.

Ross, R. and McKay, H. (1979) *Self Mutilation*. New York: Lexington Books.

Rothschild, D. (1998) 'Treating the resistant substance abuser: Harm reduction (re)emerges as sound clinical practice.' *In Session. Psychotherapy in Practice 4*, 1, 25–35.

Roy, D. (1996) 'On the ethics of euthanasia discourse.' *Journal of Palliative Care 12*, 4, 3–5.

Rudd, M., Dahm, P. and Rajab, M. (1993) 'Diagnostic comorbidity in persons with suicidal ideation and behavior.' *American Journal of Psychiatry 150*, 6, 928–934.

Rukholm, E., Bailey, P., Coutu-Wakulczyk, G. and Bailey, W. (1991) 'Needs and anxiety levels in relatives of intensive care unit patients.' *Journal of Advanced Nursing 16*, 8, 920–928.

Rustoen, T. and Hanestad, B. (1998) 'Nursing intervention to increase hope in cancer patients.' *Journal of Clinical Nursing 7*, 1, 19–27.

Saudia, T.L., Kinney, M.R., Brown, K.C. and Young, W.L. (1991) 'Health locus of control and helpfulness of prayer.' *Heart Lung 20*, 1, 60–65.

Savulescu, J. (1998) 'Two worlds apart: Religion and ethics.' *Journal of Medical Ethics 24*, 382–384.

Schmied, G. (1998) 'Praying as social action, reference, and relationship.' In J. Greer and D. Moberg (eds) *Research in the Social Scientific Study of Religion: A Research Annual.* Stamford, CT: Jai Press, pp.115–126.

Schuon, F. (1989) *Understanding Islam.* New York: Mandala.

Schwab, J. and Schwab, M. (1978) *Sociocultural Roots of Mental Illness.* London: Plenum.

Schwalbe, M. (1993) 'Goffman against postmodernism: Emotion and the reality of the self.' *Symbolic Interaction 16*, 4, 333–350.

Senay, E. and Redlich, F. (1968) 'Cultural and social factors in neuroses and psychosomatic illness.' *Social Psychiatry 3*, 89–97.

Sermeus, G. (1987) *Alternative Medicine in Europe: A Quantitative Comparison of Alternative Medicine and Patient Profiles in Nine European Countries.* Brussels: Belgian Consumers' Association.

Shah, I. (1964) *The Sufis.* London: Octagon Press.

Shah, I. (1968) *The Way of the Sufi.* London: Octagon Press.

Shah, I. (1969) *Wisdom of the Idiots.* London: Octagon Press.

Shah, I. (1971) *Thinkers of the East.* London: Octagon Press.

Shah, I. (1977) *Neglected Aspects of Sufi Study.* London: Octagon Press.

Shah, I. (1978) *A Veiled Gazelle.* London: The Octagon Press.

Shah, I. (1983) *Learning how to Learn.* London: Octagon Press.

Shah, I. (1990) *Sufi Thought and Action.* London: Octagon Press.

Shilling, C. and Mellor, P. (1998) 'Durkheim, morality and modernity: Collective effervescence, homo duplex and the sources of moral action.' *British Journal of Sociology 49*, 2, 193–209.

Sims, A. (1994) '"Psyche" – spirit as well as mind?' *British Journal of Psychiatry 165*, 441–446.

Smith, D. (1999) 'The civilizing process and the history of sexuality: Comparing Norbert Elias and Michael Foucault.' *Theory and Society 28*, 79–100.

Smith, S.M. (1972) 'Paranormal effects on enzyme activity.' *Human Dimensions 1*, 15–19.

Smolin, D. (1995) 'Praying for baby Rena: Religious liberty, medical futility, and miracles.' *Seton Hall Law Review 25*, 3, 960–996.

Soeken, K. and Carson, V. (1987) 'Responding to the spiritual needs of the chronically ill.' *Nursing Clinics of North America 22*, 3, 603–611.

Solfin, J. (1984) 'Mental healing.' In S. Krippner (ed) *Advances in Parapsychological Research.* Jefferson NC: McFarland, pp.31–63.

Solomon, G. (1987) 'Psychoneuroimmunology: Interactions between central nervous system and immune system.' *Journal of Neuroscience Research 18*, 1–9.

Sonneck, G. and Wagner, R. (1996) 'Suicide and burnout of physicians.' *Omega – Journal of Death and Dying 33*, 3, 255–263.

Sowell, R. and Misener, T. (1997) 'Decisions to have a baby by HIV-infected women.' *Western Journal of Nursing Research 19*, 1, 56–70.

Stacey, M. (1991) *The Sociology of Health and Healing.* London: Routledge.

Starrett, G. (1995) 'The hexis of interpretation: Islam and the body in the Egyptian popular school.' *American Ethnologist 22*, 4, 953–969.

Starrin, B., Larsson, G., Brenner, S., Levi, L. and Petterson, I. (1990) 'Structural changes, ill health, and mortality in Sweden, 1963–1983: A macroaggregated study.' *International Journal of Health Service 20*, 1, 27–42.

Steffen, V. (1993) 'Alcoholism and soul-surgery. Disease concepts and metaphors in the Minnesota Model.' *Folk 35*, 127–146.

Stein, M., Keller, S. and Schleifer, S. (1985) 'Stress and neuro-immodulation: The role of depression and neuroendocrine function.' *Journal of Immunology 135*, 827–833.

Stephens, R.J., Hopwood, P., Girling, D.J. and Machin, D. (1997) 'Randomized trials with quality of life endpoints: Are doctors' ratings of patients' physical symptoms interchangeable with patients' self-ratings?' *Quality of Life Research 6*, 3, 225–236.

Strauss, A. and Corbin, J. (1990) *Basics of Qualitative Research: Grounded Theory Procedures and Techniques.* Newbury Park CA: Sage.

Streib, H. (1999) 'Off road religion? A narrative approach to fundamentalist and occult orientations of adolescents.' *Journal of Adolescence 22*, 255–267.

Suarez, M., Raffaelli, M. and O'Leary, A. (1996) 'Use of folk healing practices by HIV-infected Hispanics living in the United States.' *AIDS Care 8*, 6, 683–690.

Sutton, T. and Murphy, S. (1989) 'Stressors and patterns of coping in renal transplant patients.' *Nursing Research 38*, 1, 46–49.

Tammelleo, A. (1986) '"Spiritual" nursing care: Liability issue. Case in point: Baumgartner v. First Church of Christ (490 N.E.2d 1319-IL).' *Regan Reports on Nursing Law 27*, 1, 4.

Tavolaro, K. (1991) 'Effectively and efficiently protecting children in faith healing cases: A proposed statutory revision for state intervention.' *Medicine and Law 10*, 4, 311–325.

Thomas, S. (1989) 'Spirituality: An essential dimension in the treatment of hypertension.' *Holistic Nursing Practitioner 3*, 3, 47–55.

Tinsley, H.E. and Eldredge, B. (1995) 'Psychological benefits of leisure participation: A taxonomy of leisure activities based on their need-gratifying properties.' *Journal of Counselling Psychology 42*, 2, 123–132.

Tix, A. and Frazier, P. (1998) 'The use of religious coping during stressful life events: Main effects, moderation, and mediation.' *Jounral of Consulting Clinical Psychology 66*, 2, 411–422.

Tsouypoulos, N. (1994) 'Postmodernist theory and the physician–patient relationship.' *Theoretical Medicine 15*, 267–275.

Turner, T. (1995) 'Social body and embodied subject: Bodiliness, subjectivity, and sociality among the Kayapo.' *Cultural Anthropologist 10*, 2, 143–170.

van der Geest, S. (1994) 'Christ as a pharmacist: Medical symbols in German devotion.' *Social Science and Medicine 39*, 5, 727–732.

van Leeuwen, E. and Kimsma, G. (1997) 'Philosophy of medical practice: A discursive approach.' *Theoretical Medicine 18*, 19–22.

van Manen, M. (1998) 'Modalities of body experience in illness and health.' *Qualitative Health Research 8*, 1, 7–24.

Van Ness, P. (1999) 'Religion and public health.' *Journal of Religion and Health 38*, 1, 15–26.

VandeCreek, L. (1998) 'The parish clergy's ministry of prayer with hospitalized parishioners.' *Journal of Psychology and Theology 26*, 2, 197–203.

VandeCreek, L., Rogers, E. and Lester, J. (1999) 'Use of alternative therapies among breast cancer out patients compared with the general population.' *Alternative Therapies 5*, 1, 71–76.

Vanderpool, H. and Levin, J. (1990) 'Religion and medicine. How are they related?' *Journal of Religion and Health 29*, 1, 9–20.

Varela, F. (1979) *Principles of Biological Autonomy.* New York: North Holland Press.

Vaskilampi, T. (1990) 'The role of alternative medicine: The Finnish experience.' *Complementary Medical Research 4*, 2, 23–27.

Verma, R. and Keswani, N. (1974) 'The physiological concepts of Unani medicine.' In N. Keswani (ed) *The Science of Medicine and Physiological Concepts in Ancient and Medieval India.* New Delhi: All-India Institute of Medical Sciences.

Visser, J. (1990) 'Alternative medicine in the Netherlands.' *Complementary Medical Research 4*, 2, 28–31.

Vogt, E. (1960) 'On the concepts of structure and process in cultural anthropology.' *American Anthropologist 62*, 18–33.

Wallulis, J. (1994) 'The complexity of bodily feeling.' *Human Studies 27*, 373–380.

Walrond-Skinner, S. (1998) 'The function and role of forgiveness in working with couples and families: Clearing the ground.' *Journal of Family Therapy 20*, 1, 3–19.

Walter, T. and Davie, G. (1998) 'The religiosity of women in the modern West.' *British Journal of Sociology 49*, 4, 640–660.

Walters, P. (1999) 'The doctrine of informed consent: A tale of two cultures and two legal traditions.' *Issues in Law and Medicine 14*, 4, 357–373.

Warde, A. (1994) 'Consumption, identity-formation and uncertainty.' *Sociology 28*, 4, 877–898.

Warner-Robbins, C. and Christiana, N. (1989) 'The spiritual needs of persons with AIDS.' *Family and Community Health 12*, 2, 43–51.

Waterhouse, R. (1993) 'The inverted gaze.' In D. Morgan and S. Scott (eds) *Body Matters*. Brighton: Falmer Press, pp.105–121.

Weber, M. (1964) *The Sociology of Religion*. Boston: Beacon Press.

Weinstein, M. (1974) 'Allocation of subjects in medical experiments.' *New England Journal of Medicine 291*, 1278–1285.

White, G. and Gillett, J. (1994) 'Reading the muscular body: A critical decoding of advertisements in Flex magazine.' *Sociology of Sport Journal 11*, 18–39.

Wiesing, U. (1994) 'Style and responsibility: Medicine in postmodernity.' *Theoretical Medicine 15*, 277–290.

Wirth, D. (1993) 'Implementing spiritual healing in modern medical practice.' *Advances 9*, 4, 69–82.

Wirth, D. (1995) 'The significance of belief and expectancy within the spiritual healing encounter.' *Social Science and Medicine 41*, 2, 249–260.

Wirth, D. and Cram, J. (1997) 'Multisite surface electromyography and complementary healing intervention: A comparative analysis.' *Journal of Alternative and Complementary Medicine 3*, 4, 493–502.

Wirth, D., Brenlan, D., Levine, R. and Rodriguez, C. (1993) 'The effect of complementary healing therapy on post-operative pain after surgical removal of impacted third molar teeth.' *Complementary Therapies on Medicine 1*, 133–138.

Wirth, D., Chang, R., Eidelman, W. and Paxton, J. (1996a) 'Haematological indicators of complementary healing intervention.' *Complementary Therapies in Medicine 4*, 14–20.

Wirth, D., Richardson, J. and Eidelman, W. (1996b) 'Wound healing and complementary therapies: A review.' *Journal of Alternative and Complementary Medicine 2*, 4, 493–502.

Wood, C. (1989) 'The physical nature of energy in the human organism.' *Holistic Medicine 4*, 63–66.

Worthington, E., Kurusu, T., McCullough, M. and Sandage, S. (1996) 'Empirical research on religion and psychotherapeutic processes and outcomes: A 10-year review and research prospectus.' *Psychological Bulletin 119*, 3, 448–487.

Wuthnow, S. (1997) 'Healing touch controversies.' *Journal of Religion and Health 36*, 3, 221–229.

Zborowski, M. (1952) 'Cultural components in responses to pain.' *Journal of Social Issues 4*, 16–30.

Zigmond, A. and Snaith, R. (1983) 'The hospital anxiety and depression scale.' *Acta Psychiatrica Scandanavica 67*, 361–370.

Zigmond, D. (1987) 'Three types of encounter in the healing arts: Dialogue, dialectic, and didacticism.' *Holistic Medicine 2*, 69–81.

Zola, I. (1966) 'Culture and symptoms: An analysis of patients' presenting complaints.' *American Sociological Review 31*, 615–629.

Subject Index

Author
Index

Albrecht, G. 106
Aldridge, D. 10, 11, 13, 16, 19,
  20, 21, 24, 25, 31, 35, 51,
  57, 62, 65, 68, 71, 78, 79,
  85, 86, 88, 90, 91, 93,
  102, 103, 110, 112, 122,
  129, 131, 133, 137, 139,
  145, 148, 154, 156, 158,
  159, 175, 181, 188, 193
Aldridge, D. and Pietroni, P. 156,
  188
Aldridge, D. and Rossiter, J. 154
Alter, J. 72, 73
Anderson, J.O. 105, 106
Angeletti, L., Agrimi, U., Curia,
  C., French, D. and
  Mariani-Constantini, R. 61,
  62
Aponte, H. 49, 148
Appleby, L. 113, 129
Armstrong, D. 106
Ashby, J. and Lenhart, R. 162
Astin, J. 91
Aylwin, S., Durand, S. and
  Wilson, K. 87

Baker Eddy, M. 171
Bartholome, W.G. 59
Baszanger, I. 195
Bateson, G. 14, 25, 26, 46, 47,
  53, 60, 86, 88, 92, 115,
  122, 131, 132, 139
Bearon, L. and Koenig, H. 164
Beer, S. 131
Belcher, A., Dettmore, D. and
  Holzemer, S. 163
Benedikt, M. 118
Benor, D. 15, 43, 91, 152, 168,
  196
Benson, H. 95
Berger, P. 60
Bergmark, K. 135, 167
Biddle, S. 101
Bienenfeld, D., Koenig, H.,
  Larson, D. and Sherrill, K.
  63
Bird-David, N. 75

Bloch, J. 47, 75
Blumer, H. 86
Borman, P. and Dixon, D. 28,
  37, 39
Bourdieu, P. 79, 103, 107
Bourjolly, J. 150
Boutell, K. and Bozett, F. 158
Boyd, J. 37, 40, 41, 42
Brenner, M. 113
Brewster Smith, M. 99, 104
Brown, C. 153, 154, 182
Brown, C. and Sheldon, M. 146,
  153, 182
Browner, C. 14
Bullis, R. 183
Burkhardt, M. 158
Burkhardt, R. and Kienle, G.
  188
Burkitt, I. 118
Burns, P. 166
Burston, D. 153
Buxton, M., Smith, D. and
  Seymour, R. 167
Byrd, R. 91, 167, 168

Calhoun, B., Reitman, J. and
  Hoeldtke, N. 59
Campbell, C. 59
Canale, J., White, R. and Kelly,
  K. 49, 148
Carey, G. 16
Carr, E. and Morris, T. 35
Carroll, S. 167
Carson, V. and Green, H. 164
Cassell, E. 190
Cavanaugh, M. 146, 147
Chandler, C., Holden, J. and
  Kolander, C. 28, 37
Chang, B., Noonan, A. and
  Tennstedt, S. 35, 164
Charmaz, K. 92
Chatters, L., Levin, J. and
  Ellison, G. 68
Chatters, L. and Taylor, R. 164
Clark, F., Carlson, M., Zemke,
  R., Frank, G., Patterson, K.,
  Ennevor, B.,
  Rankinmartinez, A.,
  Hobson, L., Crandall, J.,
  Mandel, D. and Lipson, L.
  35
Clark, J. and Dawson, L. 158
Cohen, J. 153
Collipp, P. 167

Compton, M. 61, 62
Conrad, N. 158
Consoli, A. 49
Conway, K. 110
Cooke, M. 164
Courtenay, A. 177
Crombez, J.C. and Dubreuco,
  J.L. 166
Crossley, N. 103
Csordas, T. 12, 22, 23, 60, 80,
  145
Cunningham, A. and Edmonds,
  C. 162
Cunningham, J., Sobell, L. and
  Sobell, M. 123
Cupitt, D. 61, 72, 136
Cutter, C. and Cutter, H. 129

Dallos, R. and Aldridge, D. 154
Davis, N.J. and Robinson, R.V.
  166
Dawson, L. 76
Dawson, P.J. 165
Decker 56
Dienstfrey, H. 143, 153, 196
Dillon, K. and Baker, K. 156
Dillon, M.C. 110
Dixon, M. 146, 156, 182
Dohrenwend, B. and
  Dohrenwend, B. 85
Dossey, B. 158, 167, 172
Dossey, L. 16, 91, 140, 141,
  146, 147, 149, 152, 153,
  169, 192
Downer, S., Cody, M.,
  McCluskey, P., Wilson, P.,
  Arnott, S., Lister, T. and
  Slevin, M. 165
Doyle, D. 27, 34, 35, 56, 68
Dreyfus, H. 104
Duckro, P. and Magaletta, P.
  149, 169
Dull, V. and Skokan, L. 154
Durkheim, E. 60, 128, 199
Duvall, N. 99

Eisenbach-Stagl, I. 116, 167
Eisenberg, L. 156
Eliade, M. 178
Elias, P. 113
Emblen, J. 27, 34, 35, 37, 66
Engebretson, J. 145
Erikson, K. 128, 129
Estes, J.W. 166